Diagnosis and Treatment of Hearing Impairment in Children

Second Edition

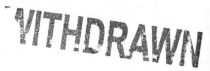

A Singular Audiology Text
Jeffrey L. Danhauer, PhD
Audiology Editor

Diagnosis and Treatment of Hearing Impairment in Children

Second Edition

Dennis G. Pappas Sr, MD

Pappas Ear Clinic
Birmingham, Alabama

SINGULAR PUBLISHING GROUP, INC.
SAN DIEGO · LONDON

Singular Publishing Group, Inc.
401 West "A" Street, Suite 325
San Diego, California 92101-7904

Singular Publishing Ltd.
19 Compton Terrace
London, N1 2UN, UK

©1998 Singular Publishing Group, Inc.

Singular Publishing Group, Inc., publishes textbooks, clinical manuals, clinical reference books, journals, videos, and multimedia materials on speech-language pathology, audiology, otorhinolaryngology, special education, early childhood, aging, occupational therapy, physical therapy, rehabilitation, counseling, mental health, and voice. For your convenience, our entire catalog can be accessed on our website at **http//www.singpub.com**. Our mission to provide you with materials to meet the daily challenges of the everchanging health care/educational environment will remain on course if we are in touch with you. In that spirit, we welcome your feedback on our products. Please telephone (**1-800-521-8545**), fax (**1-800-774-8398**), or e-mail (**singpub@mail.cerfnet.com**) your comments and requests to us.

Typeset in 10/12 Palatino by So Cal Graphics
Printed in the United States of America by Bang Printing

Library of Congress Cataloging-in-Publication Data
Pappas, Dennis G. (Dennis George), 1931–
    Diagnosis and treatment of hearing impairment in children / Dennis G. Pappas, Sr. — 2nd ed.
       p.   cm — (A Singular audiology text)
    Includes bibliographical references and index.
    ISBN 1-56593-865-8 (soft cover : alk. paper)
    1. Hearing disorders in children.   I. Title. II. Series.
    [DNLM: 1. Hearing Loss, Sensorineural—in infancy & childhood.
    2. Hearing Loss, Sensorineural—diagnosis.   3. Hearing Loss.
    Sensorineural—therapy.   WV 271 P218d 1997]
    RF291.5.C45P37   1997
    618.92' 0978—dc21
 DNLM/DLC
for Library of Congress   98-5580
                                            CIP

Contents

Preface

The current book is a successor to the previous book of 1985 and includes a reprinting of some of the classic studies from the first book. Much of the material in this book is entirely new, since, during the past decade, a considerable amount has been discovered about the prevention, diagnosis, and treatment of hearing impairment in children. Namely, considerable progress has been made in prevention of hearing loss due to influenza, the knowledge of hereditary hearing loss, the almost complete eradication of Rubella, and technological advances both in diagnosis (improved computer imaging) and in treatment (hearing aids and cochlear implants).

The first chapter of this monograph briefly focuses on the anatomy of the hearing mechanism. In this section we attempt to provide for integrated otologic, audiologic background understanding of the diseases, and conditions that cause congenital and acquired hearing loss of early childhood, for physicians, deaf educators, and parents.

In treatment of the child with sensorineural hearing loss, time is of the essence, and it is our attempt to convey to the reader those evaluations that are applicable to expeditious patient diagnosis. The chapters pursuing the causes of hearing disorders (Fundamentals of Inheritance, Hearing Loss Associated With Perinatal Infections) evaluate and discuss the various disorders causing congenital hearing loss. The scope of the book is expanded to include such topics that may affect the child with sensorineural hearing loss. These subjects include serous otitis media, congenital cholesteatoma, autoimmune inner ear disease, perilymphatic fistula, ototoxic drugs, and noise trauma.

The goal of infant hearing screening is to detect all children with hearing loss. Once identified, children can access opportunities that will allow them to lead normal lives in a communication-dependent world. Thus, the first step in caring for children with a sensorineural hearing loss is identification. Much has been written recently on this subject. We summarize the significant tests of today. Emphasis in a spoken language development program should always be on comprehension and conceptual development—activities that relate to cognition and language. Dan Ling conveys the opportunities for the child to learn the significance of events in everyday life and the language that relates to them.

The practice of pediatric cochlear implantation has grown at an exceptional pace since the publication of this book 13 years ago. Chapter 9 (Cochlear Implants) has been written to help satisfy the quest for knowledge about implantation in young children and to provide specific details about various aspects of implants.

In this book we emphasize specific subjects and techniques with which we have had experience. In 1978, a foundation and a parent-infant program (ECHO) was created (by the author) for the diagnosis and treatment of hearing impairment in children. To date over 700 children who are hearing-impaired and their families have been studied, evaluated, and helped through the ECHO program. This book represents the distillation of knowledge, skill, and experience gained in the course of such a practice.

This book should be an important guide for many otolaryngologists, audiologists, teachers, speech-language pathologists, psychologists, and other professionals working with children who are hearing-impaired and their families.

1

Overview of the Hearing Mechanism

It is of the highest importance in the art of detection to be able to recognize out of a number of facts which are incidental and which vital. Otherwise your energy and attention must be dissipated instead of being concentrated.

The Reigate Squires
Sherlock Holmes

Historically speaking, the development of this enlightened consideration for the population who are hearing-impaired is a relatively recent phenomenon. The development of a philosophy of education of so-called deaf persons has progressed very slowly. Although references to the "deaf" are scattered throughout the recorded history of all human cultures, social acceptance of this disability, let alone social awareness of the special educational needs of those who are hearing-impaired, is still the exception rather than the rule. The existence of a critical or sensitive learning period for language development is now widely accepted. This learning must occur early in life to avoid greater social, educational, and psychological disadvantages. The implications of this for the child who is hearing-impaired are obvious when the malady is diagnosed and attended in later years.

The responsiveness of the normally hearing baby to sound, and particularly to the human voice, is well-recognized by the mother. Indeed, it is the mother who often identifies her baby as having hearing impairment in the very early months of life. She makes this diagnosis based on the baby's lack of response to sound. It has been said that such clinical observations have an accuracy rate of 25% and, thus, they indicate high risk for hearing loss. Even so, there is often a long delay before hearing impairment is confirmed, amplification secured, and habilitation initiated. Reasons for such a delay include physicians' lack of awareness of the signs of hearing impairment and the psychological, emotional, social, and educational problems that ensue. Also responsible for such delays is the lack of timing of many audiologists in behavioral, or objective, testing and their inability to identify developmental milestones in hearing in the infant or young child. Identification of significant hearing loss in infancy should be accepted as a goal by those involved in this aspect of health care.

MAGNITUDE OF HEARING IMPAIRMENT

Estimates of the prevalence of permanent moderate to severe bilateral sensorineural hearing loss (SNHL) fall between 0.5 and 1 per 1000 live births; this range may be an underestimate in developing countries.[1,2] It has been further estimated that by age 6 years, the prevalence may increase to 1.5 to 2 per 1000 children.

Old statistics show the prevalence of hearing loss in the neonatal intensive care units (NICUs)[3] to have been approximately 2% of newborns. New statistics of hearing loss show 1:174 to have hearing impairment.[4]

COMMUNICATION STRATEGY

The ability to hear, listen, and communicate is developed by reflex in normal children. This is not so for the child with severe to profound hearing loss, who is characterized by a developmental failure in perceptual and linguistic skills. These children suffer not only educationally, but also psychologically.

Language is needed to develop communication skills, whether through an auditory or other modality. Deficits in this area occur at an early developmental age (by 3 years). Therefore, the following are essential:

1. Early identification of hearing impairment in infants and children.
2. Medical evaluation by the physician to determine etiology and ongoing monitoring for progression of hearing loss.
3. Provision of a sound philosophy and strategy of hearing aid amplification, regardless of the mode of education.
4. Early educational options for the child who is hearing-impaired to maximize the patient's residual hearing.

Understanding these basic concepts is especially important when dealing with children who have sensorineural hearing loss (SNHL). Once a child is identified as having SNHL, amplification with hearing aids should be provided immediately. In addition, within 2 weeks after identification, the patient and family should be initiated into a habilitation program that aims at developing a child's residual hearing and language skills. There are several methods for training children who are hearing-impaired, including the use of hearing alone (auditory), visual (speechreading), and the use of signs or fingerspelling, or both, with speech (total communication). The use of multiple-channel cochlear implants has become an important addition to habilitation. Regardless of the method used, the development of speech is an invaluable asset to the child who is hearing-impaired.

The term "deaf-mute" is to be avoided to describe children or adults with profound bilateral SNHL, because so many of them learn to speak after proper instruction, and so many have partial hearing restored with cochlear implants.

CHARACTERISTICS OF SPEECH SOUNDS: TERMINOLOGY *

Modern technology has permitted detailed study of the speech patterns used in spoken language. In English, there are about 40 different speech sounds. The sounds are combined in distinct ways to create the patterns we recognize as words. Speech patterns tend to differ from one locality to

*This section contributed by Daniel Ling, Ph.D.

another and form what are commonly called "local dialects." Most children spontaneously learn to use speech sounds in the same way as their peers and the adults in and around the home. This is not, however, the case with many children who are hearing-impaired. Spoken language is normally learned through hearing and, to the extent that children with SNHL cannot hear certain sounds, they fail to learn how to produce them. How such children talk depends largely on how they hear. Indeed, without very special help in learning to talk, the speech of children with SNHL reflects the degraded spoken language patterns that are audible to them. In this section, we shall briefly define the different speech patterns of English and describe their acoustic properties.

Just as solid objects have three dimensions—height, width, and depth—so do sounds have three dimensions—intensity, frequency, and duration. The intensity of a sound is perceived as its loudness, its frequency as its pitch, and its duration as its length. Intensity is measured in units called decibels (dB). The level at which normally hearing young people can just detect sounds is defined as 0 (zero) dB. The levels of speech in everyday conversation at a distance of 2 yards average about 60 dB and a gunshot at the same distance would be over 100 dB. Frequency is measured in hertz (Hz). When something makes a sound by vibrating backward and forward at a rate of 100 times a second, it is said to have a frequency of 100 Hz. This low frequency sound can be heard in men's voices when their vocal cords are vibrating 100 times a second. The duration of speech sounds is measured in milliseconds (ms). The shortest sounds of speech, sounds like p, t, and k, may be no more than 20 ms long, about as short as the shutter speed of a camera when the light is poor. These three dimensions constantly change in running speech. When a given speech sound is produced in running speech, it tends to be modified by the sounds that are adjacent to it. This process is known as coarticulation.

There are seven major aspects of speech: vocalization (voice), prosody, vowels and diphthongs, consonants differing in manner of production, consonants differing in place of production, consonants differing in voicing characteristics and, finally, consonant clusters, or blends.

Vocalization (voice) is produced when the vocal cords (situated in the larynx) are brought together and made to vibrate by the breath stream from the lungs, much as the lips can be made to vibrate when "blowing a raspberry." The ability to produce the relatively loud, low-pitched sounds of speech through vocalization is important for three major reasons: first, voice helps to carry speech over large distances; second, some speech sounds are normally produced with voice; and third, the way people use their voices tells the listener a lot about a talker's intentions in speaking and even about their underlying feelings. The fact that we can communicate in whispers, however, shows that while vocalization skills are desirable in speech, they are not truly essential.

Prosody is made up of variations in the intensity, frequency, and duration of voice patterns that hold our sentences and discourse together. We use prosody to stress (emphasize) words or phrases as we speak. Because it serves to clarify the meaning of what is said, prosody is linguistically important. Intonation patterns rise to indicate a question, fall when we make a statement, or vary in particular ways when we express doubt. We use prosody (particularly intonation and stress) to tell our listeners which of the ideas we are expressing are new or particularly important. Prosody also indicates speakers' moods and feelings toward their listeners. Think about how many ways there are to say the word "hello" and you will realize that prosody tells your listeners whether you are pleased to see them or have little interest in them.

Vowels and diphthongs are normally voiced. Different vowels are formed as the space between the larynx and the lips changes shape and causes movement of the air passing through this space to vibrate. This space, known as the vocal tract, resonates in different ways according to the length of the vocal tract and the way that the tongue, lips, and cheeks constrict the tract's cross-sectional area at different points in the throat (pharynx) and mouth. Several resonances (called formants) occur in the vocal tract as voicing or whispering sets the air in the vocal tract into motion. These formants vary in pitch according to the way each vowel is formed. Two formants are sufficient to identify each of the vowels; the one with the lowest frequency (the first formant—F1) and the one with the next highest frequency (the second formant—F2). The first formants of the vowels range from about 300 to 800 Hz and the second formants from about 800 to 2800 Hz. The second formants of vowels, made with the tongue at the back of the mouth, like /oo/ as in shoe, are found in the low frequency range, and those formed when the tongue is in the front of the mouth, like /ee/ as in she, are found in the higher frequencies. The second formant is the most important resonance in all vowels and is, in general, the hardest for children with SNHL to hear. Diphthongs are formed when two vowels join to make a particular sound (as in the words cow and eye). There are about 12 vowels and 4–5 diphthongs used in most English dialects. They are contained in the sentence: *Who would know more of art must learn and then take his ease again (+ my and how).*

Consonants differing in manner of production include nasals, which are made in the nose like /m/ and have the lowest frequencies of speech, and fricatives, which make a hissing sound like /s/ or /f/ and have the highest frequencies of speech. The types of sound that lie in the middle range of frequencies include the semi-vowels like /w/, the liquids (laterals) /l/ and /r/, the plosives like /p/, /t/, /k/, and the affricates, like /ch/ as in cheese. Manner of production can be differentiated mainly by acoustic cues that occur in the low frequencies.

Consonants differing in place of production are sounds like /p/, /t/, and /k/ that are made at different places (namely the front, middle, and back) of the mouth. Perception of the high-frequency energy of these consonants (from 2000 Hz up) is required to differentiate acoustic cues on place of production. Because children with SNHL tend to have the poorest hearing for high frequencies, they frequently have difficulty hearing and producing distinctions based on place of production.

Consonants differing in voicing characteristics are sounds such as /p/ and /b/. In /pa/, the plosive is made without voice by suddenly releasing the breath, but with /ba/, vocalization and breath release occur simultaneously. To detect the presence and absence of voicing in consonants, one needs to hear the harmonics of voice, which are most salient in the low frequencies.

Consonant clusters (blends) occur in words such as brown, black, and street. Consonant clusters occur in various parts of the speech frequency range.

To check whether children can detect speech sounds over the whole frequency range, one can determine how they respond to the six sounds /m/, /oo/, /ah/, /ee/, /sh/, and /sss/. These are the sounds of the Ling Six Sound Test. To identify a sound requires that any given speech sound is distinct from all others. For the child who hears normally, speech and language development follows a fairly predictable course, as shown in Table 1–1. Children with SNHL may not, unless aided very effectively from early infancy, learn spoken language skills so naturally. When children with SNHL cannot under any circumstances hear sounds, they can usually be helped to perceive and produce them through the use of other sensory modalities, namely vision and touch.

ANATOMY AND PHYSIOLOGY OF HEARING AND BALANCE

Terrence Schneiderman, MD

The general framework of the ear must be regarded as a pyramidal bony structure (temporal bone) in which the organs of hearing and balance are contained. The hearing portion is composed of three parts (the outer ear, the middle ear, and the inner ear) which perform very different functions (Fig 1–1).

Table 1–1. Stages in Development of Speech Processing

Menyuk[5] divided the development of speech processing abilities in children into the following four periods, which indicate that language acquisition occurs within a short time period; grammatical speech begins before 18 months and is complete by the age of 3 to 3.5 years. In this short span of time, an intricate competence of adult language must emerge.

1. **Infancy to 1 year:** An increasing ability to discriminate between speech sound and context. Actually, from 8 to 18 months a child can discriminate between second syllable consonant contrast (Example: puddle, puzzle) and rising versus falling intonation (Example: huho, hello). This ability depends on the child's acquiring the understanding that the perceived acoustic difference can provide a symbol for an object (that is, to name it), and that names can act as references, which can then be communicated socially.[6]

2. **1 to 4 years:** Period of rapid vocabulary growth and marked improvement in articulation (ages 3 to 4). Association of learning nonsense syllables occurs at ages 2 to 3 years.

3. **4 to 6 years:** Ability to rhyme words (Example: bake, cake) and reconstruct segmented words; establishment of morphological rules.

4. **6 to 8 years:** Can segment sentence into words (Example: That is the boy who helped me yesterday at softball practice).

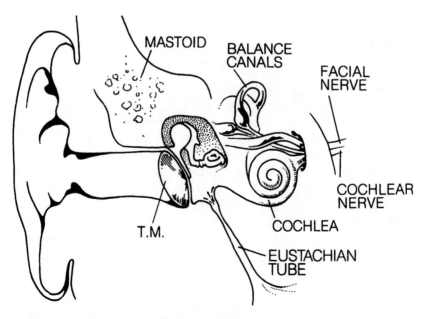

Fig 1-1.—General framework of outer, middle, and inner ear.

Outer Ear

The outer, or external, ear consists of the auricle (pinna) and a slightly curving canal (the external auditory meatus). The primary functions of the auricle are to protect the hearing mechanism and to serve as a directional funnel for sound; the function of the canal is primarily to selectively amplify the frequency range of the human voice. In humans, this amplification range approximates 4000 Hz.[7] The structural changes in the ear canal and pinna that occur during the first 3 years of postnatal growth are responsible for major alterations in the pattern of frequency sensitivity.[8] For example, the small neonate auricle and ear canal tend to produce resonance at a higher frequency than in the adult;[9] on the other hand, the ear canal of the neonate is more compliant than the adult canal and may produce less frequency resonance.[10]

In the adult, the length of the canal, one third of which is formed by a cartilage and two thirds by bone, is about 25 mm. It varies in diameter from 4 to 10 mm. The cartilaginous portion is covered by thick, hairless skin that contains glands that secrete cerumen, or wax. The purpose of this wax is to provide lubrication to protect the canal skin and to prevent the introduction of foreign bodies, such as dust, into the eardrum. The bony portion of the canal is covered by a thin, tender skin that is devoid of oil or sweat glands.

Middle Ear

The middle ear, or tympanic cavity, contains the sound-pressure transformer mechanism, the tympanic segment of the facial nerve, and a complex of vessels and nerves. The tympanic cleft is housed in the temporal bone between the tympanic membrane laterally and the otic capsule (osseous labyrinth) medially. The tegmen, or roof, of the middle ear is a thin plate of bone separating the cleft from the middle cranial fossa. The bone-covered jugular bulb forms the floor of the middle ear. The epitympanic recess is a space defined medially by the facial nerve canal and the lateral semicircular canal, laterally by the scutum, superiorly by the tegmen tympani, and posteriorly by the incudal fossa. The middle ear cleft communicates with the mastoid antrum via the aditus and antrum in the posterior-superior wall of the epitympanum recess.

The sound-pressure transformer mechanism of the middle ear consists of the tympanic membrane and the three auditory ossicles (malleus, incus, and stapes). The tympanic membrane forms the wall separating the external auditory canal from the middle ear. The outer layer of the tympanic membrane is composed of a thin skin that is continuous with the skin of the external auditory canal. The middle layer is elastic and the inner layer is continuous with the lining of the tympanic cavity. It is concave-shaped, with a diameter ranging from 8-10 mm. When viewed with an otoscope, the normal eardrum appears transparent and pearly-gray in color. Near the upper margin of the tympanic membrane, a bony protuberance (short process) of the malleus is visible on examination. An alteration in the appearance of this projection may indicate the presence of a middle ear effusion. A fold extends forward and backward from the protuberance, separating the three-layered tympanic membrane (pars tensa) from an upper, very thick, flaccid small area that is devoid of an elastic layer (pars flaccida) (Fig 1–2).

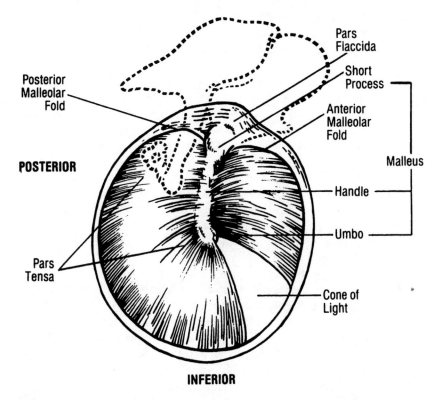

Fig 1-2.—Normal appearance of the tympanic membrane and its important landmarks. Note that a greater proportion of the malleus and incus are located above the superior edge of the bony external auditory canal and cannot be visualized by otoscopic examination. Transparency of the tympanic membrane is a normal variation and includes the ability to visualize the incudostapedial joint posterior to the handle of the malleus.

The malleus is the most lateral ossicle and is firmly imbedded in the middle fibrous layer of the tympanic membrane. The three parts of the malleus are the head, neck, and long process. The incus also consists of three parts. The body articulates with the head of the malleus within the epitympanic recess. The short process rests in the fossa incudis. The long process articulates with the head (capitulum) of the stapes. The stapes bone is shaped like a stirrup and also consists of three parts: the previously mentioned capitulum, the two stapedial crura, and a footplate, which is attached by the annular ligament to the margin of the oval window. The stapedius muscle tendon inserts along the posterior crus. Contraction of the muscle serves to place tension on the ossicular chain. The stapedial branch of the facial nerve innervates this muscle. The tensor tympani muscle originates in the roof of the eustachian tube and is four times longer than the stapedius muscle. The tendon spans the space from the cochleariform process to insert onto the medial aspect of the long process of the malleus (manubrium). The trigeminal nerve innervates the tensor tympani muscle.

The middle ear transformer system serves to amplify sound vibrations presented to the cochlea via two mechanisms. They provide an explanation as to why air conduction hearing is of greater sensitivity than bone conduction hearing. The first includes the lever system of the malleus-incus complex. The arm of the incus (long process) is shorter than the long process (manubrium) of the malleus; thus, the amount of energy applied to the stapes by the incus is greater than the originating movement of the malleus[11] (Fig 1–3). More importantly, the surface area of the tympanic membrane is much larger than that of the stapes footplate (ratio 18:1 in humans).[12] This allows the concentration of energy to localize in the cochlea (hydraulic effect).

Behind the middle ear cavity is the mastoid cavity, a "honey-comb" air cell system whose purpose is to maintain consistent air temperature and pressure. The anterior wall of the middle ear cavity contains the opening of the eustachian tube, which allows air to be introduced into the ear cavity from the lateral wall of the nasopharynx. The eustachian tube is usually closed, but during swallowing, yawning, and sneezing, it opens to permit the air pressure in the middle ear to equalize with atmospheric pressure. An individual swallows some 500 times while awake and 250 times while sleeping; therefore, middle ear pressure is constantly being equalized.

Children very frequently display eustachian tube dysfunction, which means the tube does not open when it should for the equalization of pressure between the middle ear space and the atmospheric pressure. The

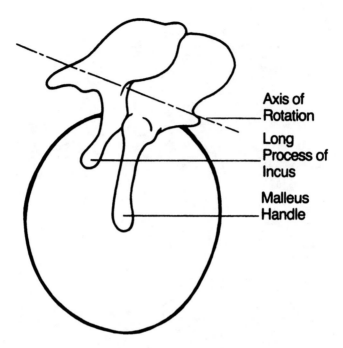

Axis of Rotation

Long Process of Incus

Malleus Handle

Fig 1-3.—Diagram showing that the force of energy at the incudostapedial joint is greater than that at its origin in the malleus: A, The malleus handle is longer than the long process of the incus (lever effect); B, the incus is rotated on the malleus about a plane of rotation, which acts as a fulcrum for the lever action about the incudostapedial joint. From G. von Békésy and W. Rosenblith. *Handbook of Experimental Psychology.* New York, NY: John Wiley and Sons, 1951: p. 102. Reprinted with permission.

most frequent reason for this dysfunction is an inflammatory reaction of the lining membrane of the eustachian tube such as that which occurs with nasal infections or allergies. Other reasons for obstruction of the tube in children include enlargement of the adenoids, developmental anomalies (such as a cleft uvula and cleft palate) and, very rarely, tumors. Such causes are more common in children than in adults because of the relative anatomical immaturity of the child's eustachian tube, which is shorter and more horizontal than that of an adult. With growth, the eustachian tube becomes longer and inclines to an angle of 40 to 45° (Fig 1–4).

Another mechanism for poor function of the child's eustachian tube rests with the immaturity of the palatal muscles. Normally, the cartilaginous portion of the eustachian tube is closed at rest. Tubal opening requires active contraction of the dilator tubae portion of the tensor veli

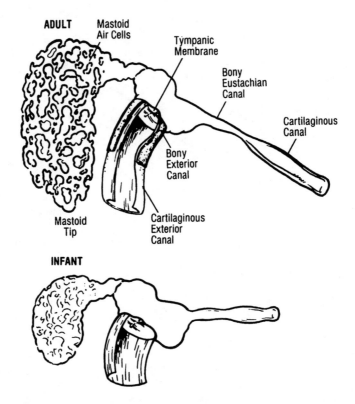

Fig 1-4. — Anatomical differences between infant and adult middle ear and external auditory canal structures. Note the lengthening, narrowing, and vertical inclination of the eustachian tube that takes place in normal development. The ossicles and inner ear structures (not shown) have reached adult size at infancy. The tympanic membrane and middle ear cavity are of the same size in infants and adults. The external auditory canal is shorter in the infant since the bony canal has not formed, but this canal is formed by age 3 years. The position of the mastoid in the infant is relatively superficial. The mastoid tip is formed by age 3 years.

palatini muscle. This portion of the muscle often does not mature until after 12 months of age.

The inability to equalize middle ear pressure results in retraction of the eardrum, a physical sense of "fullness" in the ear, and, over time, a change in the cellular makeup of the tissue in the middle ear, resulting in fluid accumulation and, most likely, a mild to moderate degree of hearing loss. With resumption of normal ventilation function, these symptoms disappear. The primary functions of the eustachian tube are to clear the middle ear secretions, impede the introduction of foreign material from the nasopharynx into the middle ear, and equalize the air pressure between the middle ear and external atmosphere.

Inner Ear

Cochlea

The sense organ of the ear is one of the highly specialized sense organs in the body. Its structures in humans are contained within the cochlea, a small, coiled tube with approximately 2.5 turns and is about 3.5 cm long. Fig 1–5, *A* is a cross-section of the cochlea illustrating the three chambers resulting from divisions made by Reissner's and basilar membranes. The interior chamber (cochlear duct, scala media, or endolymphatic duct) is triangular (Fig 1–5, B) in cross-section and contains the organ of Corti. It is the smallest of the three chambers and contains endolymph, which resembles intracellular fluid in its electrolyte composition. The larger chambers, the scala vestibuli and the scala tympani, contain perilymph, which has an electrolyte composition similar to that of extracellular fluid. The scala vestibuli is sealed at one end by the stapes footplate and the scala tympani is sealed at the base of the cochlea by the round window membrane. Fluid communicates from the scala vestibuli to the scala tympani by way of a small opening at the apex of the cochlea, the helicotrema. The endolymphatic duct is separated from the scala vestibuli by the tectorial membrane. The basilar membrane separates the endolymphatic duct from the scala tympani. Hair cells in the organ of Corti contain stereocilia, which project into the tectorial membrane, a gelatinous structure overlying the specialized hair cells (Fig 1–5, C).

Mechanism of Inner Ear Stimulation. Movement of the stapes footplate initiates a wave complex in the cochlear fluid that displaces the inner ear fluid toward the round window. This results in an outward displacement of the round window membrane. This movement of fluid is conveyed to the basilar membrane, whose elastic properties change continuously from very stiff (in the basal turn) to very soft (in the apical turn). Sound pressure in fluid produces a traveling wave, which is initially large in amplitude and decreases quickly.[13] The crest site of this traveling wave produces a displacement of the basilar membrane and is, therefore, a stimulus to this structure (place principle). The position of the maximum amplitude of the traveling wave is dependent on the frequency of the incoming sound wave (Fig 1–6, A). For example, a low frequency tone produces a maximum vibration at the apical end of the basilar membrane, whereas a high frequency tone produces a maximum vibration

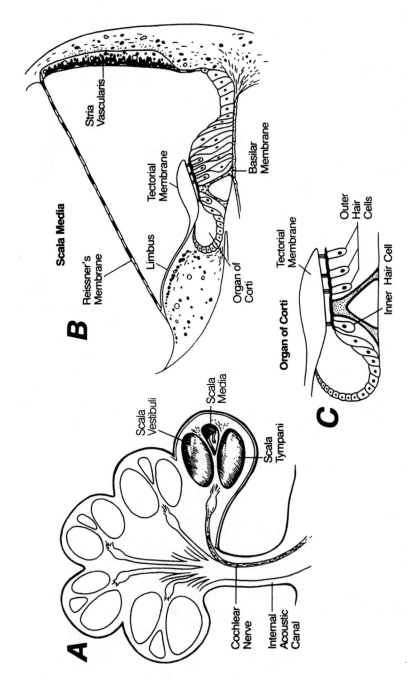

Fig 1-5. — A, Cross-section of the cochlea. B, Arrangement of the endolymphatic duct (cross-section). C, Anatomy of organ of Corti and tectorial membrane at rest.

near the basal end.[14] The range of sound frequency to which the hair cells in the cochlea are sensitive varies from 20 to 20000 Hz. Maximum upward displacement of the basilar membrane results in a shearing force between the tectorial membrane and the stereocilia of the hair cells (Fig 1–6, B). This is thought to result in alteration of membrane potentials, and, ultimately, in the depolarization of the hair cells.[14-16] These current potentials produce acoustic signals.

An interesting development, as Békésy's description of the place principle is that most animals do not begin hearing at all of their adult frequency ranges simultaneously. Rubel and co-workers[17] have hypothesized that, in many species, initial responses are elicited by low or mid-low frequencies. This hypothesis is based on the difference in developmental timing of the structural and functional processes of the cochlea and brainstem, in addition to middle ear transfer function, and the changes in the values of the place code along the cochlea during development. Responses to higher and lower frequencies, they deduced, increase as development proceeds. This principle should facilitate more accurate and optimal sound stimulations for screening the hearing of neonates.

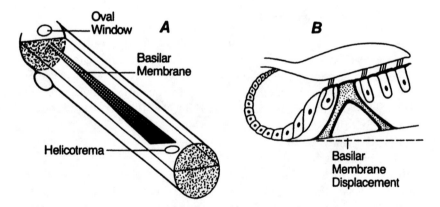

Fig 1-6.— A, Schematic diagram of the cochlea showing the basilar membrane in which the sensitive nerve cells are located. For high tones, maximum amplitude of vibrations of the basilar membrane occurs near the base, where the membrane is narrow and stiff. For low tones, maximum amplitude of vibrations occurs near the apex, where the membrane is at its widest and more flexible. B, Upward displacement of the basilar membrane resulting in a shearing force between the tectorial membrane and stereocilia of the hair cells. From G. von Békésy. Nobel Lecture, December 11, 1961. *Les Prix Nobel.* Stockholm, Imprimerie Royale Publishers, 1961. Reprinted with permission.

Auditory Nerve

Sound waves, after being transformed into nerve impulses in the cochlea, are transmitted by approximately 30 000 afferent neurofibers of the auditory division of the eighth cranial nerve to the cochlear nuclei. The cell bodies of the first order of neurons of the acoustic nerve are all contained in the spiral ganglion. At the surface of the brain, the cochlear nucleus can be seen as a swelling of the cochlear nerve. The auditory nerve divides to form the dorsal and ventral cochlear nuclei. Fibers are arranged in the auditory nerve and nuclei according to their frequency sensitivity (tonotopic distribution). Fibers that originate from the basal turn of the cochlea terminate in the most medial and dorsal areas of the ventral cochlear nucleus, while fibers from the apical turn terminate in the lateral caudal area of this nucleus. The principal nuclei of the auditory pathway, with their main connections, are shown schematically in Fig 1–7. However, it should be pointed out that the auditory pathway is more complex than just a string of relay stations on a straight line from the ear to the cortex.[18] Cross-communication of these fibers with integration of the auditory signals occurs.

The Vestibular System

The vestibular labyrinth is an important coordinating control organ for balance. It works in close relationship with the central balance system, which is composed of the brainstem, the cerebellum, and the cortex. The function of this entire balance system is to coordinate change in head position, as in turning; acceleration and deceleration, as in walking; and gravitational effects, as in positional changes from lying down on the back and turning to the side. The central nervous system (CNS), or brain, uses information from the inner ear and from the eyes, muscles, tendons, joints, and skin to regulate movements and to maintain balance and orientation. Like a computer, the cerebellum receives and processes stimuli from these various sources. It then integrates them to coordinate movements and body posture.

The sensation of motion rarely enters consciousness. Therefore, there is no simple method (such as use of pure tone thresholds for assessing hearing) of testing balance function. For this reason, clinicians must rely on reflex reactions to determine how the balance system is functioning. In this regard, the most significant reflexes arise from the labyrinth. From this portion of the inner ear, the reflexes are relayed through the brainstem, ending in the eyes (vestibulo-ocular reflex or VOR).

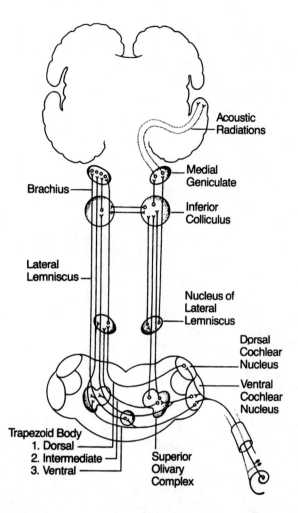

Fig 1-7. — The central auditory pathways. From RW Baloh. *Dizziness, Hearing Loss, and Tinnitus; The Essentials of Neurology.* Philadelphia, Pa: FA Davis, 1984. Reprinted with Permission.

Anatomy

The sensory structures of the vestibular organ are housed in a endo-lymph-filled membranous labyrinth which in turn is supported and housed within the contoured bony labyrinth. The latter contains peri-lymph. The sensory structures include two otolith organs and three semi-circular canals.

Each of the mechanisms of the labyrinth, or vestibular apparatus, is composed of two types of sensory receptors. One type of receptor, the crista, is located at each end of the three semicircular canals. The other type, the macule, is located in the utricle and saccule (Fig 1–8).

Each of the three bony semicircular canals lies at an angle of 90° to the others, and each responds only to changes in angular acceleration about any head axis. This reaction causes changes in neural discharge. The membranous semicircular ducts are attached by periotic tissues to the bony canals and are suspended in perilymphatic fluid. The ends of each duct originate at the utricle and return to the utricle. Each semicircular duct is dilated at one end before it joins the utricle. The dilation, the membranous ampulla, is approximately 2 mm in diameter and contains the neuroepithelium of the semicircular duct. Each ampulla contains the crista, which is made up of a group of hair cells and their supporting cells. The hairs from these cells project into the cupula, a mass of jelly-like material (glycoproteins) that acts like a hinged weather vane (or diaphragm) in the system. Inside the cupula, stereocilia and kinocilia project from the hair cells. The semicircular duct is completely blocked by the cupula at the cupulocrista junction, where the cupula bends according to the flow of endolymphatic fluid that surrounds it in the semicircular canal (Fig 1–9).

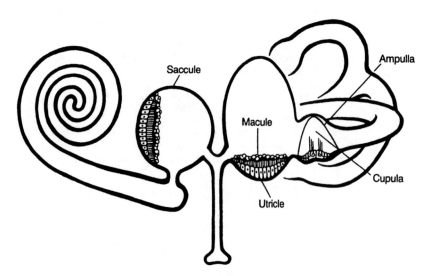

Fig 1-8.— Diagram of the membranous inner ear showing the crista of the lateral semicircular canal and the macule of the saccule and utricle. From Minnigerode and Stenger. *Spontan-und Provokations-Nystagmus.* Berlin: Springer-Verlag, 1982. Reprinted with permission.

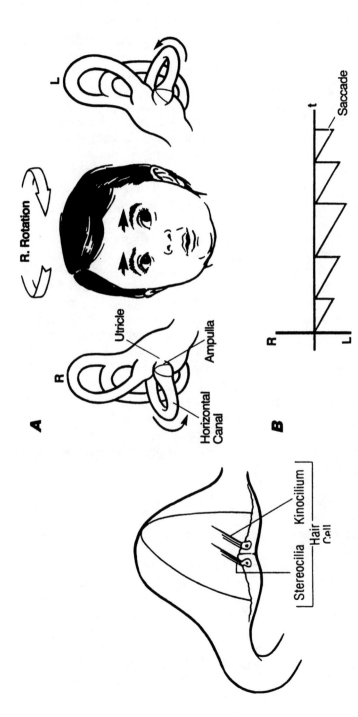

Fig 1-9. — A, Angular rotation (to the right) produces flow of endolymphatic fluid in the horizontal canal toward the cupula, and consequent cupular deviation toward the utricle. The response to this stimulus is an eye movement, or deviation, opposite to that of the rotation. B, The amplitude of the slow phase eye velocity of the horizontal eye movements will vary with the acceleration stimulus. Saccades (reset movements) are compensatory movements introduced periodically to reset the eye position. These saccades are removed by the central processor.

19

The hair cells within the crista are aligned in the direction of the kinocilia. In the horizontal canal the kinocilia are directed toward the utricle, and in the vertical canals (superior and posterior) they are directed toward the canal. Thus, a difference in directional sensitivity is produced between the horizontal and vertical canals.[19,20] In the horizontal canal, when endolymphatic flow causes cupula deflection toward the utricle, there is neural excitation in the canal and neural inhibition in the posterior and superior canals. The opposite occurs when angular head acceleration results in endolymphatic motion causing deflection of the cupula away from the utricle.

Normal end organs of the vestibular canals give a bilateral constant and equal discharge when at rest.[20,21] When the discharge rate of the two sides becomes unequal, the sensation of vertigo is experienced.

The membranous labyrinth also forms two cavities within the vestibule, the utricle and the saccule, each containing a receptor organ, or macule. The utricle, an elliptical structure, is closely associated with the duct systems of the semicircular canals. The channels (lumens) of the semicircular canal systems continue into a full circle through the cavity of the utricle. The saccule is a circular structure, closely associated with the endolymphatic duct of the auditory system. The maculae of the utricle and saccule also consist of hair cells and a gelatinous mass that in some ways resembles the cupula. However, on the surface of this gelatinous mass are pure white crystals of calcium carbonate known as otoliths (also called ear stones, otoconia, or statoconia), which make the utricle and saccule gravity-dependent organs (Fig 1–10). This property of otoliths distinguishes the macula from the cupula, which has the same specific gravity as the surrounding fluids and is not subject to gravitational force.

When the head is erect, the utricular macula is horizontally positioned, and the saccular macula is vertical. The macula of the utricle responds to linear acceleration and deceleration in a horizontal plane. Although the function of the saccule is unknown, it seems to respond to vibration and vertical acceleration.

The fluid system of the membranous labyrinth is the same one that is continuous with the fluid system of the endolymphatic duct. The cupula and the maculae of the labyrinth could be considered transducers in which the mechanical energy of the stimulus (endolymphatic fluid movement in the system by motion or gravity, or both) is transformed into an electrical signal. This electrical signal triggers the liberation of energy, which initiates the nerve impulse in the vestibular nerve.

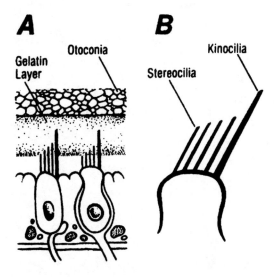

Fig 1-10.— A, Anatomy of the macule. B, Mechanism of hair cell activation with a gravitational change.

Vestibulo-Ocular Reflex

Nerve impulses from the labyrinth proceed through the vestibular nerve to the brainstem, then to four vestibular nuclei. Some nerve fibers are conveyed directly to the cerebellum. There is selective distribution of nerve fibers to the four nuclei from the cristae of the semicircular canals and the maculae of the utricle and saccule. Impulses from the four nuclei are then conveyed through the hindbrain (through the spinal column to all muscles, tendons, and joints) to the cerebellum and through the forebrain to the nuclei that initiate movements of the eyes. It is this reflex, the VOR, that is measured by vestibular testing. The presenting sign of this testing is the response of nystagmus, a slow movement of the eyes that originates in the labyrinth as a result of a stimulus, and a compensatory fast jerk of the eye that has its origin in the cortex of the brain (Fig 1–11). Portions of the cortex control all nuclei in the brainstem that control eye movements.

Internal Auditory Canal and Facial Nerve

The internal auditory canal (IAC) transmits the seventh and eighth cranial nerves from the brainstem. The eighth cranial nerve consists of the

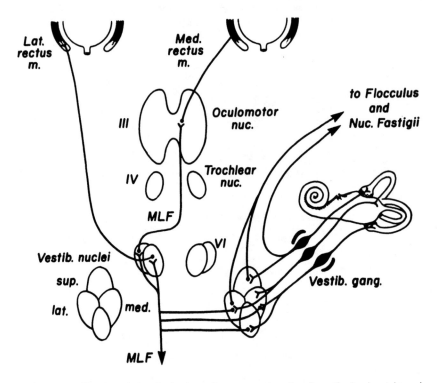

Fig 1-11. — Simple pathway for horizontal nystagmus. Impulses from the horizontal canal are conveyed to the vestibular nuclei (VN). Ascending branches cross the midline of the brainstem to the para-abducens and abducens nuclei (VI). The abducens nucleus gives rise to the abducens nerve, which supplies the lateral rectus muscle (LR). The cells of the para-abducens nucleus, or reticular formation, give rise to the axons that cross the midline shortly after their origin to ascend in the medial longitudinal fasciculus (MLF) to that part of the oculomotor nuclei that supplies the medial rectus muscle (MR).

cochlear and vestibular division. A complex relationship exists between the nerves as they come from the brainstem to the most lateral aspect (fundus) of the IAC. Initially, the vestibular nerve is superior to the cochlear nerve as it courses laterally from the cerebellopontine angle (CPA) into the IAC. It rotates posteriorly and splits into the superior and inferior vestibular nerve on its way to the labyrinth. The superior vestibular nerve innervates the para superior (superior and lateral semicircular canals and utricle). The inferior vestibular nerve innervates the pars inferior (posterior semicircular canal and saccule).

The cochlear nerve, initially representing the inferior division of the eighth nerve as it leaves the brainstem, courses anteriorly to occupy the anterior-inferior aspect of the fundus.

The seventh cranial nerve (facial nerve) is closely associated with the auditory nerve. Although the facial nerve is not responsible for auditory transmission, the establishment of the normal function of this nerve is very important in determining the site-of-lesion in certain disorders. For this reason, an understanding of anatomy and function of this nerve, especially the acoustic reflex, is essential in evaluating the auditory system.

The facial nerve occupies the anterior superior portion within the internal auditory canal and remains anterior to the superior vestibular nerve and superior to the cochlear nerve. As the facial nerve courses laterally and leaves the IAC, it separates from the eighth nerve and passes superior to the transverse crest and anterior to a vertical crest of bone known as "Bill's bar." After leaving the IAC, the facial nerve lies separately within a bony canal (fallopian canal). This segment (labyrinthine segment) lies superior to the cochlea and vestibule and extends to its geniculate ganglion (internal genu, or "knee"). At this point, the nerve makes a sharp posterior turn and starts the tympanic segment. The nerve courses superior to the oval window and medial to the malleus and incus. The facial nerve then makes a second turn inferiorly (external genu) just under the lateral semicircular canal. This marks the beginning of the mastoid segment, which exits the temporal bone from the stylomastoid foramen.

The temporal bone houses four branches of the facial nerve: the greater and lesser superficial petrosal nerves arising from the geniculate ganglion, the nerve to the muscle which arises from the mastoid segment as it crosses the middle ear, and the chorda tympani, which leaves the facial nerve above the stylomastoid foramen.

The Stapedius Reflex

The nerve fibers responsible for the muscle reflex pathway project from each ear to the ipsilateral and contralateral brainstem so that intense sound to one ear produces a simultaneous reflex in both ears. This occurs when a sound stimulus of 70 to 90 dB above threshold hearing causes a response contraction of the muscle.

The stapedial reflex arc[22] consists of sound conveyance to the hair cells in the organ of Corti and neural stimulation of the primary afferent auditory neurons, ipsilateral secondary neurons in the ventral cochlear nucleus, bilateral tertiary neurons in the superior olivary nucleus, and bilateral motor neurons in the facial nucleus (Fig 1–12).

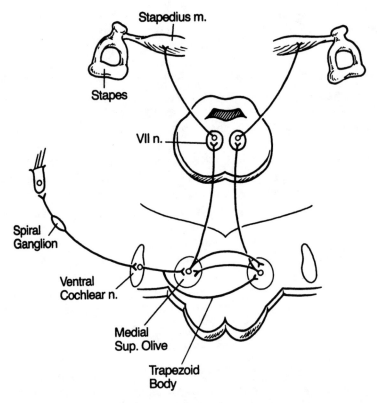

Fig 1-12.— Central connections of acoustic reflex. From R.W. Baloh. *Dizziness, Hearing Loss, and Tinnitus: The Essentials of Neurology*. Philadelphia, Pa: F.A. Davis, 1984. Reprinted with permission.

EMBRYOLOGICAL NOTES

Auditory dysfunction can usually be attributed to some form of abnormal structure. An understanding of the development of the normal ear is essential in understanding the effects of aberrant development in the abnormal ear. Anomalies of the inner ear will result in SNHL, which requires educational habilitation. Anomalies of the auricle, external auditory canal, or middle ear (or all of these) cause conductive hearing loss in most cases, and rehabilitation by the use of hearing aids, surgery, or both will provide normal hearing.

To understand the types of anomalies that occur, a knowledge of the timing of the embryonic development of the ear is necessary. In cases in which an exogenous injury, caused by a drug or virus, is the cause of the anomaly, it may be possible to determine at what point in gestation the injury occurred. Sando and Wood[23, pp291-292] have suggested the following injury–gestation time schedule.

In the third week of fetal development, the eustachian tube and tympanic cavity start to form as an outpouching from the lining of the developing pharynx.

During the second month, this outpouching comes into contact with the developing external auditory canal to form the tympanic membrane. This development is complete at 4 months of gestation. The ossicles start to form (from cartilage) and begin to ossify at 16 weeks, reaching adult form at 35 weeks. By 30 weeks of gestation, the tympanic cavity is complete. The main cavity of the mastoid process, the antrum, appears in the 23rd week of fetal life. Air cells begin to develop in the bony structure from the antrum in the 35th week, and the development of the tympanic cavity is not completed until after birth.

From these superficial highlights, it is obvious that the most important developments occur during the first 4 months of gestation. Minor remodeling of these formations, especially that of the auricle, may not be complete until the seventh month of gestation. Major defects of the outer and middle ear will be manifested in the first trimester; minor deformities can appear later, up until the seventh month. The inner ear begins its development at 3 weeks from a separate and different tissue. It arises from nerve tissue that first forms a platelike structure (auditory placode) alongside the posterior brain and later forms a vesicle (sac). It should really be considered an extension of the brain. From one end of the vesicle, three extensions arise, each forming a semicircular canal. The superior canal forms first; the horizontal last. This process is completed by the seventh week. During the formation of the semicircular canal, the utricle develops in association with the canals and the saccule becomes demarcated from the rest of the vesicle. The anterior portion of the saccule extends into a spiral growth forming the endolymphatic duct. By the 10th week of gestation, this spiral growth has developed 2¾ turns and has reached its full length.

During the eighth week, the scala vestibuli and scala tympani appear from surrounding tissue at the base of the cochlea. By the end of the fourth month of pregnancy, these structures have extended beside the endolymphatic duct and coalesced to form the helicotrema. This entire membranous structure is then surrounded by a cartilaginous capsule that ossifies to form bone. By the fifth month of gestation, the organ of Corti is fully developed.

Of particular interest are cases in which the embryo has been exposed to a well-defined chemical agent at a specific stage of its development. A situation in which a mother had taken tablets equivalent to 100 to 200 mg of thalidomide approximately 25 days after conception was described by Jorgensen and co-workers.[24] The ingestion of this chemical resulted in the mother giving birth to a child with aplasias (failure of development) of both inner ears. The embryonic vesicle would have been the only structure present at that period. Generally in such cases, other structural anomalies are found, including abnormalities of the middle and external ears. In a series of cases of external auditory canal atresia, Naunton and Valvassori[25] demonstrated that these deformities are sometimes accompanied by defects in the inner ear (12%). This would suggest that inner ear defects must be investigated when defects of the outer ear are found.

Jackler and Luxford[26] described a classification of inner ear maldevelopment. Arrest in the maturational continuum of inner ear development resulted in various inner ear defects, depending on when the arrest in embryogenesis occurred. The spectrum ranges from complete labyrinthine aplasia (Michel deformity) to normal development. Approximately 20% of patients with a congenital SNHL will have these defects found as radiographic abnormalities of the inner ear.[26]

EMPHASIS ON EARLY IDENTIFICATION AND MONITORING OF PROGRESSIVE SNHL

Numerous discussions of the progression of a SNHL are presented throughout the text. Although some cases of progressive SNHL are idiopathic, there are a number of etiological factors known to be associated with this condition. In approaching a resolution to the problem of progressive SNHL, the pathophysiology of the condition and its probable cause must first be considered (Table 1–2) since the recommendations for treatment are based on these.

Conditions that demonstrate or fail to demonstrate progression of the hearing loss are identified on the basis of repeated audiograms. However, at least 10 to 15 years of monitoring a large population of patients with progressive SNHL may be necessary to develop definitive criteria. So far, the progressiveness of impairment in SNHL is characterized by its irregularity. That is, there may be long periods of time during which hearing loss appears to become stationary, only to be followed by sudden and rapid progression. This progression may be bilaterally symmetrical or asymmetrical and involve low, mid, or high frequencies.

Table 1–2. Progressive Sensorineural Hearing Loss (SNHL) in Children*

Common Causes	Mechanisms
Hereditary delayed (including syndromes)	Hereditodegenerative chemical deficiencies, such as occur in metabolic syndromes
Virus, congenital	Reactivation of dormant virus; immune response
Bacterial meningitis	Calcium deposits in cochlea; mechanical or chemical, as in endolymphatic hydrops
Syphilis	Continual destruction by organism; mechanical or chemical, as in endolymphatic hydrops
Space-occupying lesions	Acoustic neuromas, meningiomas, vascular anomalies, congenital cholesteatomas
Congenital hereditary	Recessive, dominant, sex-linked (hearing loss at birth)
Birth injuries	Low birth weight, perinatal asphyxia, hyperbilirubinemia (underlying combinations of conditions, such as acidosis, sepsis, drugs, and hypoglycemia may cause neurological damage)
Head trauma	Temporal bone fracture; labyrinthine concussion
Ototoxicity (progression may followdrug administration for months, then should stablize) sound trauma	Aminoglycosides antibiotics, diuretics (eg, ethacrynic acid, furosemide), aspirin, antiprotozal agents

*Excluding perilymphatic fistulae and autoimmune inner ear disease. Progression of a hearing loss should be suspected in all children with a SNHL.

REFERENCES

1. Chan KH. Sensorineural hearing loss in children: classification and evaluation. *Otol Clin North Am.* 1994;27:473-486.
2. Brookhouser PE. *Sensorineural Hearing Loss, Pediatric Otolaryngology for the General Otolaryngologist.* Hotaling, AJ, Stankiewicz, JA, eds. New York, NY: Igaku-Shoin; 1996:263-277.
3. Schulman-Galambos C, Galambos R. Brain stem evoked response audiometry in newborn hearing screening. *Arch Otolaryngol.* 1979;105:86-90.
4. Davis A, Wood S. The epidemiology of childhood hearing impairment: factors relevant to planning of services. *Br J Audiol.* 1992;26:77-90.
5. Menyuk P. Effect of persistent otitis media on language development. *Ann Otol Rhinol Laryngol.* 1980;89(suppl 68):257-263.

6. Ling D, Neinhuys TG. The deaf child. Habilitation with and without a cochlear implant. *Ann Otol Rhinol Laryngol.*1983;92:593-598.
7. Calvert DR, Silverman SR. Speech and its production. In: *Speech and Deafness.* Washington, DC: Alexander Graham Bell Association for the Deaf; 1975:64-68.
8. Manley GA. The hearing mechanisms. In: Hinchcliffe, R, ed. *Hearing and Balance in the Elderly.* Edinburgh: Churchill Livingstone; 1983:44-73.
9. Shaw EAG. The external ear. In: Keidel WD, Neff WD, eds. *Handbook of Sensory Physiology, Auditory System,* Vol I. New York, NY: Springer-Verlag; 1974: 455-490.
10. Saunders JC, Kaltenback JA, Relkin EM. The structural and functional development of the outer and middle ear. In: Romand R, Marty R, eds. *Development of Auditory and Vestibular Systems,* New York, NY: Academic Press; 1983:3-25.
11. von Békésy G. *Experiments in Hearing.* New York, NY McGraw-Hill; 1960:102.
12. Wever EG, Lawrence M. *Physiological Acoustics.* Princeton, NJ: Princeton University Press; 1954:69-114.
13. von Békésy G. Concerning the pleasures of observing, and the mechanic of the inner ear. In: *Les Prix Nobel.* Stockholm: Imprimerie Royale Publishers; 1961:184-208.
14. Davis H. A model for transducer action in the cochlea. *Cold Spring Harbor Symp Quant Biol.* 1965;30:181-90.
15. Honrubia V, Strelioff D, Sitko ST. Physiological basis of cochlear transduction and sensitivity. *Ann Otol Rhinol Laryngol.* 1976;85:697-710.
16. Strelioff D, Haas G, Honrubia V. Sound-induced electrical impedance changes in the guinea pig cochlea. *J Acoust Soc Am.* 1972;51:617-620.
17. Rubel EW, Born DE, Deitch JS, Durham, D. Recent advances toward understanding auditory system development. In: Berlin C, ed. *Hearing Science.* San Diego, Ca: College-Hill Press; 1984;109-157.
18. Moller AR. Physiology of the ear. In: Bluestone C, Stool SE eds. *Pediatric Otology,* Vol I. Philadelphia, Pa: WB Saunders; 1983;112-138.
19. Lowenstein OE, Wërsall J. A functional interpretation of the electron microscopic structure of the sensory hairs in the cristae of the elasmobranch *Raja clavata* in terms of directional sensitivity. *Nature.* 1959;184:1807-1808.
20. Baloh RW, Honrubia V. Vestibular function: An overview. *Clinical Neurophysiology of the Vestibular System.* Philadelphia, Pa: FA Davis; 1979;1-21.
21. Hoagland H. Impulses from sensory nerves of catfish. *Proc Natl Acad Sci.* 1932;18:701-704.
22. Baloh RW. Dizziness, *Hearing Loss and Tinnitus: The Essentials of Neurology.* Philadelphia, Pa: FA Davis; 1984:51-52.
23. Sando I, Wood RP II. Congenital middle ear anomalies. *Otol Clin North Am.* 1971;4:291-318.
24. Jorgensen MB, Kristinsen HK, Buch NH. Thalidomide-induced aplasia of the inner ear. *Ann Otol Rhinol Laryngol.* 1970;79:1095-1101.
25. Naunton RF, Valvassori GE. Inner ear anomalies: their association with atresia. *Laryngoscope.* 1968;78:1041-1049.
26. Jackler RK, Luxford WM, House WR. Congenital malformations of the inner ear: a classification based on embryogenesis. *Laryngoscope.* 1987;97(suppl 40):2-14.

CHAPTER

2

Pursuing the Causes
of Hearing Disorders

*Detection is, or ought to be, an exact science,
and should be treated in the same cold and
unemotional manner.*

The Sign of Four
Sherlock Holmes

Acceptable pediatric health care should include the detection and prevention of auditory diseases and malfunctions. This should be accomplished at the earliest age possible, since the evaluation, habilitation, and education of the young patient who is hearing-impaired depend on early treatment. To achieve these minimum requirements demands astuteness and subtlety in the design and adaptation of the physician's clinical approach to obtaining the medical history and executing the physical examination.

Sixty percent of differential diagnoses are made during otolaryngological evaluation history taking. Therefore, subsequent diagnostic accuracy depends on a thorough medical history, including the most complete family history as possible. The physician who develops the art of history taking has a great advantage over the one who depends primarily on physical findings and laboratory tests. Information obtained from the determination of cause may be very useful in the management of a patient.

NEED FOR A THOROUGH HISTORY AND PHYSICAL EXAMINATION

Genetic Information Gathering

When a SNHL has been positively diagnosed in one offspring, genetic counseling is indicated for family planning. To be considered are concerns such as the increased risk of having subsequent children with SNHL or other genetic disorders, future genetic counseling for the hearing-impaired, and the options available to a high-risk couple.

Parental Anxiety Amelioration

Minimizing parental anxiety and guilt can be a great contribution to the well-being of a family; parents seem relieved when a cause is determined. This knowledge includes insight into the probability of normal couples having youngsters with hearing impairment and the diminished risk of a similar viral disease causing a second child to be born with a hearing impairment.

Typically, parents who have a dominant genetic feature have already accepted that hearing loss and other defects may be present. This is not so in families where there is no evidence of a white forelock, wide-set eyes, and so on. In dealing with the recessive cause of genetic SNHL, the physician should try to alleviate anxiety by conveying to the parents the fact that the gene defect comes from both the mother and the father. Usually, one can explain recessiveness on the basis that there are five or six existing defective genes for hearing in all individuals, and should individuals having the same defective genes marry, the chances are high that a child will inherit a SNHL. Such an explanation would tend to alleviate anxiety that one or the other parent is responsible for a hearing loss.

Diagnosis of Other Conditions

Other defects that may be associated with hearing impairment can be anticipated and the appropriate outcomes can be expected. These include: failing vision in Usher's syndrome, thyroid dysfunction in Pendred's syndrome, and drop attacks with cardiac disorders in the Jervell and Lange-Nielsen syndrome. In other words, there is a high incidence of other organ involvement in children with SNHL, and the appropriate examinations are necessary to make a diagnosis and define concomitant systemic abnormalities.

Medical or Surgical Intervention

Some causes of hearing impairment are amenable to treatment, such as syphilis (penicillin and cortisone), the fluctuating hearing loss of meningitis (cortisone), autoimmune inner ear disease (cortisone), inner ear defects with fistulae (repair),[1,2] and kidney transplant in Alport's syndrome.

Determination of the Predicted Course of the Hearing Loss

Progression of the hearing loss can be anticipated when the loss is due to certain causes. In meningitis, for example, some fluctuation or progression is expected, especially in patients with mild to moderate hearing loss.[3] This is important information for amplification, as well as for parental edification.

Preventive Measures

Patients with inner ear defects are at high risk for sudden or progressive hearing loss due to perilymph fistulae and should be restricted from activities that would "stress" their ears.[2]

Habilitation

A rational approach to habilitative techniques can be used for the child. Pure auditory-verbal approaches can be made when the hearing is normal at birth followed by a progressive hearing loss during the first years of life. When "symptomatic" cytomegalovirus (CMV) disease has caused a total hearing loss and central damage with mental retardation, it is very unlikely that the child will be able to learn language by an auditory-verbal approach; therefore, an alternative mode of communication must be chosen.

THE HISTORY IS TAKEN, NOT GIVEN

A probing history must be extracted, or taken, from the patient. For example, rather than asking, "Does anyone in your family have hearing problems?" ask instead, "Has anyone in your family had ear surgery, worn hearing aids, learned sign language, or had any trouble hearing at all?" or, "Are there siblings with learning problems?" Questions of this nature yield more specific information related to the patient's family history. This includes family histories of nephritis (Alport's syndrome) in other children or young adult family members, retinitis pigmentosa (RP) (Usher's syndrome), and syndromic phenomena. The obvious should be stressed here: The paternal, as well as the maternal, history should be a part of every patient's medical history. Significant facts related to the patient's own medical history that may suggest an associated hearing impairment may be elicited in this same fashion (Tables 2–1 and 2–2).

There are two specific areas in which the physician must be knowledgeable to obtain an efficacious history and physical examination:

1. The examiner must have a thorough knowledge of high-risk factors for nerve hearing loss and how these factors operate. For example, there may be no clear relationship between any single birth injury high-risk factor (hyperbilirubinemia, asphyxia, and so forth) and hearing loss. The specific levels of bilirubin sufficient to cause hearing damage are difficult to determine. Infants with a bilirubin concentration of 35 mg/dl may have no hearing loss, whereas others with a level less than 12 mg/dl may have hearing impairment. There is, of course, the possibility that other high-risk factors were present simultaneously and combined in various ways to produce hearing loss. Low birth weight (LBW) is associated with complications of hyperbilirubinemia; asphyxia is associated with acidosis, sepsis, or hypoglycemia (or all three); and a combination of these may damage peripheral and central neurological tissue. Therefore, multiple factors can support the diagnosis of birth injury high-risk factors as the cause of hearing loss. There is a high incidence of brain damage with this group of risk factors.[5,6] In addition to hearing loss, other common manifestations of CNS injury must be sought. These include cerebral palsy, mental retardation,

Table 2–1. Determination of Risk Factors in Infants and Children — Speech and Hearing Checklist*

Hearing[†]	Age	Speech: Does the Child...[†]
Does the baby react to your voice even when he or she can't see you?	3 months	Babble to self (Even babies who are deaf babble)
Does he or she turn to the source of the sound?	6 months	Babble approximations of consonant sounds: m, n, p, b, k, g, t, and d
Does he or she acknowledge or react to environmental sounds: dog barking, telephone ringing, someone's voice, his or her own name?	7–10 months	Repeat sounds others make
Does he or she point to familiar objects or people when asked questions such as: Find the ball? Does he or she respond to different sounds?	11–15 months	Say "mama" and "dada" appropriately; use first words with meaning and know three words
Can the child point to body parts on request without the questioner making a gesture?	18 months	Repeat words others say: "Go bye-bye"; "Want cookie"
Can he or she follow simple commands: "Get your hat and give it to Daddy." "Bring me your ball." Can he or she point to features of pictures in a book on request?	2 years	Use a variety of everyday words heard in home environment; refer to self by name; use short, telegraphic sentences
Does he or she recognize meaningful sounds: telephone; car door closing when family member arrives home?	2 years	Say or sing short rhymes or songs
Does he or she respond appropriately when you call him or her from another room?	2 years	Understand and use simple verbs, pronouns, prepositions and adjectives, such as go, me, in, and big; use complete sentences some of the time

* Reprinted with permission of the Alexander Graham Bell Association for the Deaf, Washington, DC.
†If "No" to any of these, refer to hearing testing; no child is too young to be tested.

Table 2–2. Speech and Hearing Milestones*

3 months:
> Jumps (startles) to sudden loud sounds.
> Stirs from sleep when there is a loud noise.
> Stops sucking when there is a sudden new sound.
> Smiles at mother.
> Has a special cry when hungry.
> Coos when fed and dry.
> Laughs.
> Holds head up straight while lying on stomach.

6 months:
> Turns in general direction of a new or sudden sound.
> Usually stops crying when mother talks to him or her.
> Enjoys a musical toy.
> Reaches out to be picked up by someone in the family.
> Seems to enjoy making sounds with voice like "baba" and "ooh,ooh."
> Chuckles, gurgles, or laughs when playing.
> Makes happy sound when sees is going to be fed.
> Rolls over, either from back to front or from front to back.

9 months:
> Responds to his or her name, to "No" and "bye-bye."
> Knows if a person's voice sounds friendly or angry.
> Looks directly at a new sound or voice.
> Plays peek-a-boo.
> Imitates speech but doesn't use real words.
> Seems to be using "own words" to name things.
> Makes a lot more and different sounds than a few months ago.
> Sits well without any help.

12 months:
> Uses a variety of consonant sounds (eg: g, m, n, d) when he or she babbles.
> Strings sounds together and changes his or her voice inflections to sound as if he or she is asking a question.
> Uses his or her voice to get another's attention.
> Says words or groups of sounds which sound like words.
> Is able to stand while holding onto a chair or other support.

*From P.E. Brookhouser.[4] Reprinted with permission.

epilepsy, aphasia, and behavioral disorders.[7] Signs of these conditions may add objective support to the presumptive diagnosis of a birth injury high-risk factor.

2. The physician must be cognizant of all clinical features of any disease that may result in a hearing loss. The following case history illustrates this point. The example is that of rubella; although this disease has been almost eradicated, there is an occasional case that emerges, indicating the need for a knowledge of the clinical features of the disease.

An unimmunized mother contracted rubella in the first trimester. She was given injections (probably gamma globulin [GG]) and developed no signs of rubella. The delivery was complicated by "atrophy" of the umbilical cord and oxygen was administered to the baby for 4 days. When the child was evaluated years later, cerebral palsy was diagnosed and a mild to moderate bilateral hearing loss was identified. The probable cause of the hearing loss was either rubella or hypoxia. The child had been immunized against rubella at the age of 15 months. At age 5 years his agglutination titer was 0.6, his mother's 2.2. It is known that rubella infections contracted after birth appear to give long-term immunity with high antibody production. It has also been determined that prenatal rubella does not produce high antibody titers, and these prenatal antibodies tend to disappear. The diagnosis of congenital rubella could be excluded if the rubella titer was not high, which would indicate that the titer did not respond to the rubella vaccine at age 15 months.

The characteristics of progressive hearing loss vary with different diseases. Hearing loss tends to remain stable if caused by anoxia or hypoxia at birth; progression of hearing loss is known to occur in cases of rubella, especially in the first years following birth.[8] Returning to the preceding clinical history:

At age 8 years, this child developed a left facial paralysis that was thought to be secondary to a cholesteatoma (intact tympanic membrane), which was removed. However, as there was no erosion of the facial canal apparent at surgery, it is doubtful that the cholesteatoma was the cause of the facial paralysis. The hearing of the left ear returned to previous threshold levels, but a month later a high frequency SNHL was determined to be progressive and severe in the left ear and moderate in the right ear. The patient's speech was reportedly poor during this month (Fig 2–1). Results of computerized tomography (CT) of the temporal bone structures and brain, electroencephalogram (EEG), and ophthalmological examination were all normal. Serum antibody studies, lymphocyte subpopulations, and other white cell counts (sedimentation rate, rheumatoid factor, and fluorescent treponema agglutination) were also normal. The presence of a rapidly pro-

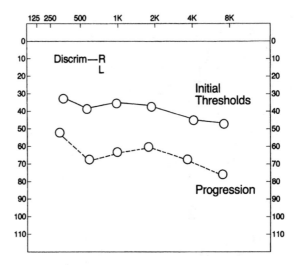

Fig 2-1.—Slow progression of hearing loss in the right ear over a 1-month period. The results for the left ear are not shown, but this ear showed a similar increased hearing threshold.

gressive hearing loss, facial paralysis, and response to treatment with dexamethasone would indicate that the patient developed an autoimmune inner ear disease, although he had been previously diagnosed as having central auditory damage due to hypoxia.

When SNHL has been identified in an infant or child, an extended historical examination is necessary to determine the cause. The extraction of a complete medical and family history in such cases probably requires more time and diagnostic skill than any other part of the evaluation; however, it may yield more useful information than any other portion of the evaluation battery. The potential benefits from a painstakingly thorough history cannot be overemphasized.

Events within the prenatal, natal, and postnatal periods are important in determining the cause of the hearing loss. Unfortunately, more often than not, the cause of the hearing loss cannot be proved by laboratory data, and the physician must rely on presumptive reasons.

Outline of Diagnostic Evaluation

The purpose of this outline is to provide the examiner with a usable guide that has been found to be the most suitable for a history assessment of patients who are hearing-impaired. The known causes of congenital and acquired hearing loss in infants and children are outlined according to prenatal, natal, and postnatal factors.

I. Prenatal evaluation with extended family history of any of the following parental factors.
   A. Ototoxic maternal medications, especially aminoglycosides,[9,10] salicylates,[11,12] or quinine[13] (which has been known since early in this century to be used as an abortifacient[14]) and chloroquine phosphate.[15,16]
   B. Diseases in the mother such as meningitis and, possibly, juvenile and uncontrolled diabetes,[17,18] which are known to cause hearing loss.
   C. Maternal head injury with complications such as unconsciousness, hemorrhages, oxygen deprivation, and so forth.
   D. Immunizations to rubella.
   E. Parental drug usage, especially the possibility of drug abuse; use of teratogenic agents, such as radiation toxins; and the use of all chemicals and drugs should be elicited. The use of agents such as these by either parent could cause a hearing impairment in a child through hemolytic anemia and kernicterus as a result of hepatitis, toxic liver damage, or blood-borne sepsis.
   F. Numerous spontaneous abortions or miscarriages. These may be associated with some type of stereospecific chromosomal abnormality.
II. Natal evaluation high-risk factors: Evaluating the etiological factors responsible for irreversible damage to the cochlea and brainstem is not a simple task. According to the Joint Committee on Infant Hearing in 1990,[19] the following factors are associated most commonly with hearing loss.
   A. Genetic history of parents' families. Keep in mind that early clues may not be present. The majority of inherited hearing defects usually do not offer clues that are immediately obvious to the physician. This point is stressed because of the belief of some clinicians that, in the absence of a family history, the presence of a genetic factor is unlikely. One example of a contradiction to this fallacy is for offspring with cystic fibrosis.[20] Until the birth of the first child in a family to have this genetic manifestation, there will be no family history on either side of individuals afflicted by the condition. This is more true for rarer diseases. A hereditary hearing loss resulting from a new mutation is difficult to ascertain. In the case of hearing loss, another sibling with the same defect will confirm inheritance.

B. Congenital viral infections. A viral screen has been recommended if the neonate has failed a hearing screen.[21] The known congenital viral or infectious disorders causing hearing loss may be asymptomatic at birth (CMV, 90%; rubella, 50%; syphilis, 50%).[22]

C. LBW—less than 1500 grams (under 3.3 lbs).

D. Unconjugated bilirubin exceeding the level that indicates a blood transfusion.

E. Severe asphyxia with an arterial pH of less than 7.5 and accompanied by coma, seizures, or the need for continuous assisted ventilation, or according to the Joint Committee identification criteria, which includes infants with Apgar scores of 0-3 at 5 minutes, those who fail to initiate spontaneous respiration by 10 minutes, or those with hypotonia persisting to 2 hours of age.

F. Presence of head and neck defects.

G. Meningitis (viral before birth, bacterial after birth).

H. Ototoxic medications including, but not limited to, the aminoglycosides used for more than 5 days (eg, gentamycin, tobramycin, kanamycin, streptomycin), and loop diuretics used in combination with aminoglycosides.

I. Prolonged mechanical ventilation for a duration equal to or greater than 10 days (eg, persistent pulmonary hypertension).

J. Stigmata or other findings associated with a syndrome known to include SNHL (eg, Waardenburg or Usher's syndrome).

III. Postnatal evaluation of patient's history.

A. Parent/caregiver concern regarding hearing, speech, language, and/or developmental delay.

B. Meningitis, bacterial (still the most common cause of acquired hearing impairment).

C. Inheritance (some hereditary causes of hearing impairment may have a delayed onset or be manifested after the inner ear has developed normally), stigmata, or other findings associated with syndromes known to include SNHL (eg, Waardenburg or Usher's syndrome).

D. Head injury, especially with longitudinal or transverse fracture of the temporal bone.

E. Drugs (especially ototoxic).

F. Infections and SNHL: Number and severity of episodes of purulent otitis media or chronic otitis media followed by progressive high frequency SNHL, or fluctuating SNHL.[23] Has a diagnosis of Reye's syndrome (viral infection, aspirin intake, increased serum ammonia level) been made? Are measles and mumps associated with bilateral SNHL?

G. History of immunological disorders (in children: overly persistent bacterial or viral infections, connective tissue disease, hematological disease, glomerulonephritis). Included are children with neurodegenerative disorders such as neurofibromatosis, myoclonic epilepsy, Werdnig-Hoffman disease, Tay-Sach's disease, infantile Gaucher's disease, Niemann-Pick disease, and any infantile demyelinating neuropathy.

PHYSICAL EXAMINATION

Since it is impossible for the physician to remember all of the diagnostic signs of a hearing loss associated with syndromes, astute observation should characterize his or her physical examination of the patient. Focusing first on the general relationship and then on specific systemic features will enable the physician to circumscribe, in a logical manner, the possible cause for the hearing impairment in a child, and as a result prescribe only those laboratory tests necessary for further delineation and ultimate confirmation of a diagnosis.

The thyroid must be examined for goiter; if no evidence of such is found, further testing is not indicated unless there is a family history of SNHL and goiter. Heart sounds should be examined and the abdomen checked for organ enlargement. A funduscopic search should be done for evidence of RP or the localized pigmentation that sometimes occurs in rubella. Further careful scrutiny by the examiner may reveal gross symmetrical defects suggestive of possible SNHL or differentiating the patient from others in the same age population, thereby permitting an early projected diagnosis. For example, certain symmetrical abnormalities are related more to conductive hearing losses, while others are related more to SNHL. Therefore, the first step in the otorhinolaryngological examination of the young patient is the observation of age-determinate symmetrical relationships. This includes not only the region of the head and neck, but also the relationship of the torso to the extremities. Measurements are not necessary since astute observation can detect micro- or macrocephaly and morphological asymmetries of the torso to the extremities, fingers to hands, arms, and so forth.

At the conclusion of the examination, the physician will have inspected and assessed the entire head and neck, the body and extremities, and all of the cranial nerves of the pediatric patient as far as the age-dependent circumstances have permitted. The outline in Fig 2–2 is not complete, but is one used by the author for children in all age groups as an aid in diagnosing SNHL.

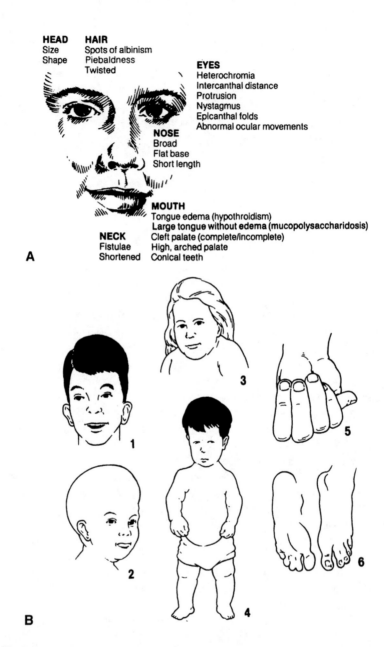

HEAD
Size
Shape

HAIR
Spots of albinism
Piebaldness
Twisted

EYES
Heterochromia
Intercanthal distance
Protrusion
Nystagmus
Epicanthal folds
Abnormal ocular movements

NOSE
Broad
Flat base
Short length

MOUTH
Tongue edema (hypothroidism)
Large tongue without edema (mucopolysaccharidosis)
Cleft palate (complete/incomplete)
High, arched palate
Conical teeth

NECK
Fistulae
Shortened

A

B

1
2
3
4
5
6

Fig 2-2.—Physical Examination: Systematic examination should start with the head and neck (A). The physician may try to differentiate systematically normal from abnormal (B). Besides making a diagnosis, prognostic information may be obtained.

Ears: Supernumerary tags, atresias, stenosis or absences, low-set (B,1), preauricular pits, auricular deformities.

Nose: Broad, flat-base, short length.

Head: Too large (B,2) or too small (associated with mental retardation). Most common known cause of microcephaly is intrauterine infection.

Hair: A white forelock (Waardenburg's syndrome) may present as a streak of white hair from the middle of the forehead or slightly off-center. A common finding and may occur as a hereditary sign without hearing loss.

Eyes: If the eyes are too close together mental retardation is more likely than when eyes are too far apart. Protrusion, epicanthal folds, congenital nystagmus, abnormal ocular movements.

Facial Appearance: Various syndromes can be associated with different facial configurations including coarse features (mucopolysaccharidosis or various storage diseases), fine facial features (William syndrome), triangular face (progeria); round face (Prader-Willi syndrome), flat face (Potter syndrome), and expressionless face (myotonic dystrophy).

Mouth: Large tongue caused by hypothyroidism may prevent mental retardation if treated early, when present with neonatal hypoglycemia, it can be lifesaving or can prevent mental retardation. Large tongue occurs with omphalocele or umbilical hernia in Beckwith-Wiedemann syndrome. Cleft palate may be an isolated finding, or it may be associated with other syndromes. A bifid uvula has same genetic implications as cleft palate.

Neck: A child with a shortened neck (B,3) is likely to have abnormalities of the vertebrae; fistulae may also be present.

Hands, Feet: A fingerlike thumb is present in congenital heart disease; the thumb sign is seen in Marfan's syndrome (B,5). Nail dysplasias, webbing of toes 2 and 3 (B,6); and broad terminal phalanges .

Stature: Use of a growth chart is necessary. If the child is below the 3rd percentile but has continued to grow, the diagnosis is most likely familial short stature. It is a significant sign if the child was in the 25th percentile, then stopped growing, and is now below the 3rd percentile. Children with short stature as a result of hypopituitarism are usually proportionately short; those with short limbs or trunk may have a skeletal dysplasia (B,4)

Skin: Neurofibromatosis associated with café au lait spots may be one of the most common genetic skin syndromes. Dark brown lentigines; albinism; hyperkeratosis; atrophy.

Renal: Progressive nephritis (Alport's syndrome), hypertension; abnormal steroidogenesis and hypogenitalism, infantile renal tubular acidosis, hyperprolinemia and ichthyosis, urticaria and amyloidosis, macrothrombocytopathia and nephritis. (Based on M. Feingold.[27] Reprinted with permission.)

Examination for Head and Neck Defects

The anatomy of the head and neck is considered for defects. Ear anomalies, associated with head and neck anomalies, may occur in the following ways[24]:

1. As a result of primary regional defect (eg, otocraniofacial syndromes).
2. Secondary to a primary defect in an area contiguous to the temporal bone (eg, craniofacial dysostosis).

3. As part of an inherited defect involving the skeletal system (eg, osteopetrosis).
4. As part of a chromosomal disorder (eg, trisomy 13-15 syndrome).

What particular defects are associated with congenital hearing loss? What physical signs are positively associated with hearing loss in infants? Unfortunately, these questions cannot be answered unequivocally. Perhaps an explanation of deformations versus malformations would aid in understanding the probability of congenital losses.

A congenital deformity is an alteration in the shape or structure of a previously normal part. Deformations arise most frequently during late fetal life. Since the most common cause of deformations is intrauterine molding, the musculoskeletal system is usually affected. The most important factor contributing to deformations is lack of fetal movements owing to, for example, small amounts of amniotic fluid. For instance, mandibular deformation can result from the mandible and shoulder being pressed sharply together for a long period of time in utero. A folded-down pinna is another example of a deformation. Deformities occur in about 2% of all newborns[25] and develop during the fetal period following organogenesis, consequently affecting intact areas. Therefore, congenital losses are less likely to be discovered with deformations than with malformations.

Malformations, which may be relatively simple or quite complex, arise during the organogenetic period of embryonic life; the later the defect is initiated, the simpler the malformation. Malformations may be minimally or maximally expressed. For example, bifid uvula is a minimal expression of a cleft palate; a completely cleft palate would be a maximally expressed malformation.

A single minor malformation occurs in 15% of all newborns. The occurrence of two minor malformations is less common, and the presence of three or more minor anomalies is distinctly unusual, occurring in approximately 1% of all newborns. It is interesting to note here that a major malformation is found in 90% of newborns found with three or more minor malformations.[26] There is clear implication that any infant or child presenting a number of minor malformations should be closely examined for a hidden major malformation.

In examining a child, it is of great importance to note if any defects present are malformations or deformations and whether they are numerous or occur in isolation.

The External Ear and Ear Canal

If a physician is to recognize an abnormal pinna, he or she must first examine it in its normal state. The pinna, or auricle, is composed of a piece of elastic cartilage with numerous convolutions covered with thin skin. The major convolutions include the helix, antihelix, tragus, antitragus, and concha. In the normal ear, the superior border of the helix is located at the level of the outer canthus of the eye, and the tragus is roughly level with the intraorbital rim.

Be watchful of a perfectly "normal" ear when there is some abnormality of the other ear. The apparently "normal" ear does not necessarily have normal hearing; the incidence of congenital middle ear anomalies in the good ear opposite a malformed one is extremely high.

Jaffe[28] has reported unilateral conductive hearing loss in children with normal-sized pinnae and unilateral absence of the superior crus. He has also reported hearing loss in patients with fused antihelix-helix, thickened, hypertrophied earlobes, a "cup" ear, and protruding pinna (Fig 2–3).

After a physician has examined many auricles, the differences between normal ears becomes striking. It is important to realize that an abnormal-appearing pinna should be viewed with suspicion rather than as a definite indication of hearing loss. Wide variation exists even in ear convolutions that are within normal limits. Differences in the shape of the pinna between individuals are so marked that European police forces use the configuration of the auricle for identification much like fingerprints are used in this country.

Abnormal Pinna. Microtia is translated literally as "small ear." Variations can range from slight to total absence of the pinna (anotia).

Atresia (closure of the external auditory canal) is generally classified into three types.[29] Type I is mild and is characterized by a small ear canal and an almost normal middle ear. Type II is of medium severity; a bony atresia plate replaces the canal and ossicular malformation is common. Type III is severe; both the ear canal and the middle ear space are small or absent.

Multiple combinations of atresia and microtia exist. Congenital middle ear problems occur in virtually all children with these abnormalities. As a rule, the milder the microtia or atresia, the less severe the anomaly, and the more easily surgical correction is achieved. SNHL has been found in 12% of the patients with congenital atresia of the outer ear.[30]

When stenosis (narrowing) of the ear canal or another defect is found, it is imperative to investigate the possibility of other malformations of the middle and inner ear systems.

Nose

Examination of the ears should be followed by examination of the nasal area for possible defects. Look for an unusually broad nose with a flat

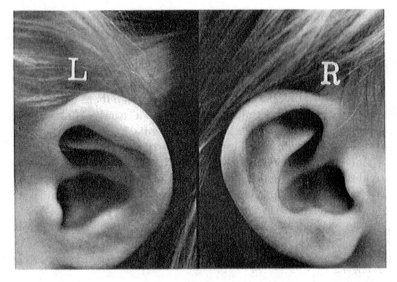

Fig 2-3. — Notice the difference in the structure of the auricle. This young patient had a mixed hearing loss in the left ear, and normal hearing in the right ear.

base and short length ("saddle nose"). This may sound like the description of the average newborn's nose, but the physician is looking for unusual proportions. Other suspicious defects of the nose are unusually small nostrils and notched alae.

Mouth

An obvious defect in this area is a cleft lip or palate. Deformities of the lip and palate are among the most common malformations. Although SNHL is not usually associated with clefts, the child with this deformity must be followed closely because of the tendency to develop chronic otitis media. The child with cleft lip or palate displays a deficiency of palate musculature, which is related primarily to the inability of the tensor veli palatini muscle to dilate the eustachian tube actively during swallowing.[31] This condition leaves the child susceptible to effusion of fluid and, as a result, various degrees of conductive hearing loss. Studies of the incidence of hearing loss in cleft palate patients indicate an average prevalence of 50%, with the loss generally being bilateral and conductive. It must be noted that the degree of severity of cleftness of the palate does not seem to have any influence on the degree of middle ear problems. Therefore, a child with a submucous cleft and bifid uvula must be followed just as closely as a child with a complete cleft.

Other possible defects of the oral cavity are edema of the tongue (indicative of hypothyroidism), large tongue without edema (mucopolysaccharidosis), high arched palate, and conical or malformed teeth (dominant onychodystrophy).

Eyes

Konigsmark and Gorlin[32] have listed over 20 hereditary diseases in which both the auditory and the visual systems are affected. It should be noted that most of these congenital problems are associated with SNHL.

Deformities of the lid are the most usual abnormalities involving the eyes. Normally, the same amount of sclera is visible on either side of the cornea. The eyelids are joined medially at the same level as the medial side of the cornea. Epicanthic folds are true vertical folds extending from the nasal fold into the upper eyelid. These folds are common in Down's syndrome and are normally present during fetal development from the third to the sixth month, disappearing by birth.[33] Occasionally, they persist for several months as a temporary, but normal, variable structure.

Fisch[33] reported another variation in eyelid configuration in which the upper lid forms an almost vertical curve at the level of the medial limit of the cornea and fuses with the lower lid (Fig 2–4). The distances of the two medial angles of the eyelids are increased by the eyelid deformity, but there is no displacement of the eyeballs. These findings were typical in a group of patients identified as having Waardenburg's syndrome, which most typically also produces numerous variations in the pigmentation of the iris (Fig 2–5).

Hair

Unusual hair texture or hairline should be regarded with suspicion. Twisted hair (pili torti) has been associated with SNHL of various degrees.

The hair in such cases may be described as dry, brittle, easily broken, or twisted. Other hair defects that may be significant are aberrant scalp hair patterning, such as piebaldness and spots of albinism.

Neck

Notable defects of the neck present at birth are branchial cleft fistulae and a mildly webbed, or shortened, neck. Goiters are symptomatic of Pendred's syndrome in association with bilateral SNHL ranging from mild to profound in degree.

Epicanthal Fold

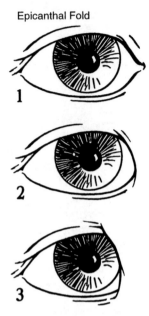

Fig 2-4.—Epicanthic folds. **1.** Normal eye in Caucasian and Negroid races. **2.** Normal structure in infant (may be temporary). **3.** True epicanthic fold; not to be confused with increased intraocular displacement of the eye.

It cannot be overemphasized that every child with an unusual auricular fold does not necessarily have an accompanying congenital hearing loss. As mentioned earlier, there is so much variation among normal individuals that it is sometimes very difficult to differentiate a normal from an abnormal pinna. Instead of attaching so much significance to a single physical finding, then, it is much better to view the whole child. Acute observation should characterize the physician's physical examination and a more than routine ear, nose, and throat examination should be done. Unusual facial or body features may suggest a syndrome as the cause of the hearing loss (Fig 2–2, A and B).

VESTIBULAR TESTING

Vestibular Function in Children

When an SNHL is present in a child, knowledge of whether or not the balance system is functioning normally enables the physician to (1) better identify and classify the cause of the SNHL, (2) differentiate motor prob-

Iris

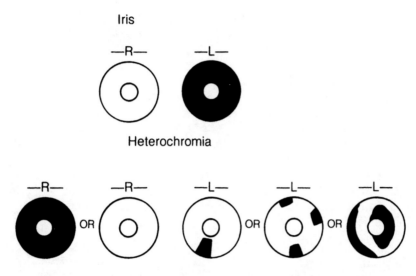

Heterochromia

Various combinations of heterochromia and/or pigmentation

Fig 2-5. — Fisch's observation of the numerous variations in the degree of pigmentation seen in Waardenburg's syndrome. (From L Fisch. Reprinted with permission.)

lems of vestibular origin from those of central origin, and (3) give insight into symptoms of dizziness or postural instability. In addition, accidents related to balance might be avoided. For example, the absence of inner ear function may result in a loss of stabilization of the patient's position while swimming in deep water. In fact, vestibular deficits are common in children with congenital or early profound SNHL.

In the habilitation process, determining that children with decreased vestibular responses have delayed motor development rather than early signs of developmental delay is important. Children with vestibular dysfunction who have a delay in the acquisition of head control, retarded motor development, and postural instability have frequently been labeled "brain damaged" or "mentally retarded." Symptoms of vestibular instability in children include easy stumbling and falling, veering to one side when crawling or walking, and inability to sit without leaning. Fine movements, such as grasping, are usually normal.

Motor delays secondary to vestibular dysfunction resolve with time and usually without treatment. The vestibular system has diffuse connections with the CNS, and central compensation will alleviate the various instabilities. This compensatory development may require months (up to 1 year) following the vestibular insult.

It is often very difficult to use conventional testing techniques to determine the cause of dizziness and loss of hearing in children. Many children will not tolerate the discomfort and possible nausea with vomiting associated with some diagnostic evaluations. Indeed, when such discomfort is accompanied by trepidation and emotional trauma, the desirability of such testing loses rank on the priority scale. As a consequence of these facts, the balance system has not been thoroughly studied in cases of congenital or acquired hearing loss in children.

It is not difficult to test cooperative children on the rotary chair (rotation or turning). In fact, most children can be made to perceive the test as a game. It is often helpful to test infants while the child is being held in the lap of its mother or an assistant. Given a reasonably cooperative patient, there is no difficulty in obtaining accurate test results using the rotary chair.

Clinical Testing

Vestibular testing in children with hearing loss includes either standard electronystagmography (ENG), especially caloric stimulation, or computerized rotary chair testing (RT).

Results of caloric stimulation in children with SNHL and vestibular damage may range from diminished activity of the labyrinth to absent responses. Abnormal vestibular function is accurately quantified with RT, since both labyrinths are stimulated simultaneously. Of these tests, caloric stimulation with alternate cool and warm water, has been the most widely used. Each labyrinth is tested separately; consequently, the function of each inner ear is elicited.

When RT is not available, some useful and clear, although nonspecific, information can be gained by simply turning the patient in a chair that will rotate. The patient is fully rotated, by hand, 10 times in 30 seconds, then brought to a sudden stop. After 5 minutes, the turns are repeated in the opposite direction. A difference of 30% in the duration of nystagmus produced by equal spins in two directions is indicative of a past or present vestibular lesion. If there is little or no nystagmus with rotation to both sides, the labyrinths are considered to be hypoactive or nonfunctioning.

When postural control was evaluated with posturography by Enbom et al,[34] the forces actuated by the feet were recorded with force of the platform equipped with strain gauges. Eighteen children, ages 12 to 16 years of age, with congenital or early acquired bilateral vestibular loss and impaired hearing were tested. Body sway velocities increased in both abnormal and normal children, but increased more significantly in children with bilateral vestibular loss when subjects stood on foam rubber. When this testing modality is not available, useful and clear, although nonspecific, information can be gained by simply using a form foam rubber platform.

Importance of Vestibular Testing for Children With SNHL

The need for vestibular testing in children with SNHL is emphasized. A differential diagnosis can be greatly elucidated in hereditary SNHL with vestibular testing. In studying 14 cases with SNHL, (9 bilateral, 5 unilateral) Oliveira and Schuknecht[35] found pathologically that bone and fibrous tissue in both cochleas and vestibular labyrinths had no more than 10% of cochlea neurons remaining. They concluded that this was a good correlation of the integrity of the sensorineural units of the lateral semicircular canal with the preservation of cochlea neurons. They then suggested that caloric tests would be useful in predicting the status of the neuronal population in the cochlea.

Caloric Tests in Children

The actual result of stimulation by a caloric irrigation is movement in the endolymph (of the lateral semicircular canal), displacing the cupula (Fig 2–6). The response of this cupula deviation is measured by the degree of nystagmus demonstrated by ENG (Fig 2–7). A variety of caloric tests are used clinically. These differ only in the volume and temperature of the water used. The objective is to have a stimulus that will evoke deviation of the cupula. One method of accomplishing this in children is to initially use threshold irrigations (30°C, 42°C) in each ear canal. If this does not produce nystagmus, ice water irrigation is begun using a stream of 5 ml over 5 seconds. The vestibular apparatus is said to be inactive if ice water does not produce nystagmus.

The younger the patient, the less readily accepted the stimulus of this test. We have been able to accomplish caloric testing on patients 3 years of age and older; it is an exception to accomplish full testing, especially in infants of age 1 year or younger. Despite the limitations of nonrotational testing, this is the test that is preferable for testing of vestibular function in infants and young children.

Computerized Rotary Chair System (Rotary Test or RT)

Angular acceleration tests (turning, rotation) have been employed in evaluating the vestibulo-ocular reflex (VOR) of the vestibular system since 1906.[36] The technology of computer science now makes it possible

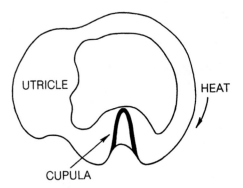

Fig 2-6.—Caloric stimulation. A warm caloric irrigation of the horizontal semicircular canal changes the specific gravity of the fluid in the canal, producing a flow toward the cupula (and utricle) and causing a slow phase of nystagmus toward the ear being stimulated. Cool water causes fluid to flow away from the cupula and a slow phase of nystagmus to the opposite ear.

to more accurately analyze responses to vestibular stimulation. The intent of this section is to provide a brief conceptual and functional description of the computerized rotary chair system to those who may not be familiar with the developments[37-39] in this test modality.

The stimulus used in rotary testing of the vestibular system is low frequency harmonic acceleration "turning" (rotation). The response to this stimulus is the motion of the eyes, which is measured at various stimulus frequencies (rotations). By computer, this response is graphed in a "response curve" that indicates the function of the vestibular system (Fig 2–8). A function of the VOR system is to stabilize the ocular line of sight with respect to the ground in the presence of a moving ocular platform. Inertial motions of the head or ocular platform are sensed by the motion organs, a set of each are located in both labyrinths. Each set consists of three angular acceleration organs (cupulae) and two linear acceleration organs (otoliths) (Chapter 1, p. 20).

On a right horizontal rotation, the endolymphatic flow in the semicircular canal is in the direction opposite to the rotation, resulting in a slow component of nystagmus (the cupula having been bent toward the utricle). The opposite endolymphatic movement occurs in the left labyrinth on right rotation (endolymph displaces the cupula away from the utricle). In accordance with Ewald's second law,[40-42] this response represents the combined effects of stimulation that excites the crista of one labyrinth and the inhibiting effect on the crista of the opposite side during rotations. This stimulation, inhibition or asymmetry information, is acquired in the very low or high frequencies of rotation. Mid-frequency range of rotation (0.2 to 10 Hz) gives symmetrical responses.[43]

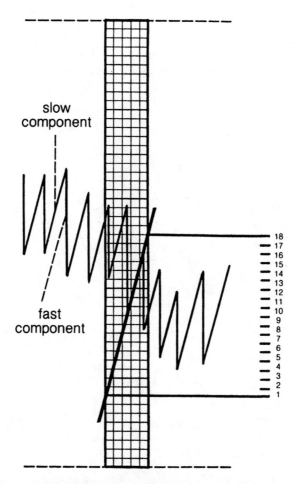

Beats of vestibular nystagmus recorded with ENG.

The velocity of the slow eye movement (degrees/sec.) is measured as above.

Fig 2-7. — Beats of vestibular nystagmus recorded with ENG. The velocity of the slow eye movement (degrees/sec) is measured as in the figure.

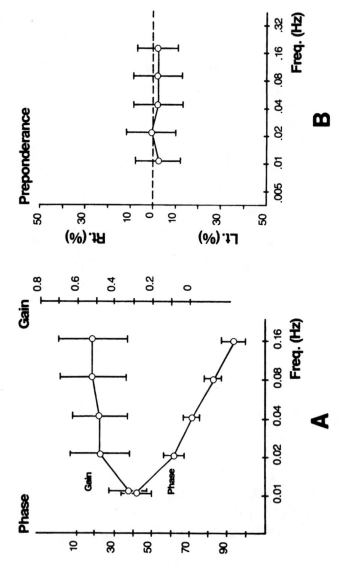

Fig 2-8.—Format for response parameters elicited in very low frequencies of rotation. Five discrete turning tests are presented (abscissa). Vertical bars for the phase parameter indicate variations for that parameter in 104 normal subjects. A, The gain parameter demonstrates normal values in these 104 subjects, but it is typically given as individual figures for each frequency of stimulation in a separate computer printout sheet. B, The response parameter preponderance. Although phase deviations are determined by the degree of frequency of stimulation in a separate computer printout sheet. B, The response parameter preponderance reflects the amount of CNS compensation following labyrinthine lesion.

CLASSIFICATION OF HEARING LOSS

The known possible causes of hearing impairment are quite numerous, but one natural distinction commonly found in the literature is between congenital hearing impairment, in which the cause of the auditory loss is presumed to have been in operation before birth, and acquired hearing impairment, in which the cause of the hearing loss supposedly occurs at or after birth. Acquired hearing loss occurring at or before birth is congenital (eg, CMV SNHL is acquired before birth and is congenital). The term "congenital hearing impairment" is understood to mean any sensorineural hearing impairment that may be either actually or potentially present at birth, regardless of whether or not such auditory loss was documented at that time. The use of the term congenital hearing impairment, moreover, is not to be restricted to or confused with hereditary causes of sensorineural hearing impairment among pediatric patients. Thus, all cases of SNHL with a genetic basis are congenital, but congenital causes of SNHL are not always genetically based (Table 2–3).

Perhaps the most significant aspect of the classification of SNHL is that both genetic and metabolic congenital factors operating before birth to produce hearing loss often manifest their effects after birth. Cases of congenital syphilis are obvious examples of this observation, but a more important illustration of such a delay is found in patients in whom hearing is normal at birth and hearing loss is manifested in later years. Other examples are the "early syndromes" and "late syndromes" of SNHL among children. The age at which "early" and "late" syndromes are separated has not been defined clearly. It is useful to consider hearing loss that emerges prior to, or during, the time of speech and language development as an early syndrome. The late syndrome case is one in which the

Table 2–3. Classification of Sensorineural Hearing Loss in Childhood

I. Congenital
   Genetic
   Nongenetic
   Inflammatory, traumatic, toxic, metabolic, neoplastic

II. Delayed
   Genetic
   Nongenetic
   Inflammatory, toxic, metabolic, neoplastic, traumatic

hearing loss emerges following the development of speech and language (Tables 2–4 and 2–5).

The classification of hearing loss is facilitated by dividing the disorder into categories of the common congenital causes. Accurate classification can be a significant aid in the evaluation of a hearing loss.

Table 2–4. Common Congenital Causes of SNHL

Cause of Hearing Loss	Audiologic Signs	Other Characteristics
Congenital, hereditary none symptomatic		
Dominant	Variance; unilateral or bilateral; usually progressive	None
Recessive	Variance; bilateral	None
Sex-linked	Severe or profound; usually bilateral.	None
Congenital, acquired		
Rubella	Variance	May involve CNS, heart, eyes
Cytomegalovirus	Variance; Asymmetrical; Progressive	May involve CNS, dental structures, liver
Congenital Syphilis	Normal at birth, low frequency onset age ±7, progressive	Speech language develops normally
Perinatal		
Neonatal Asphyxia	Variance: Worse high frequency usually stable	Subclinical or clinical CNS involvement
Hyperbilirubinemia	Variance: Worse high frequency & usually stable	Subclinical or clinical CNS involvement
Prematurity	Variance: Worse high frequency & usually stable	Subclinical or clinical CNS involvement

Typically, perinatal causes co-exist.

Table 2–5. Syndromes Causing SNHL

Cause of Hearing Loss	Audiologic Signs	Other Characteristics
Ophthalmic		
Usher syndrome	Bilateral	Retinitis pigmentosa (RP) Rare, prior age 3, RP may or may not be present 3–6. Typical after age 6.
	Type I sloping at 40–76 dB Type II Severe-profound corner audiogram	
	Type III Low frequency loss(Rare type)	
Refsum syndrome	High mid frequency sloping progressive	RP typically after age 9. late onset(after age 9), Spino-cerebellar ataxia
Alström syndrome	Progressive bilateral, flat, or sloping Late onset (age 8–9)	Retinal degeneration and optic atrophy, obesity, diabetes after age 10, Renal failure 3rd decade
Others: Hallgren syndrome Laurence-Moon-Biedl syndrome		
Renal Disease		
Alport syndrome	Progressive, bilateral, worse mid-high frequencies, onset age 8.	Hematuria at birth, nephritis with progressive renal failure
Thyroid		
Pendred syndrome	Full syndrome: Severe-profound at birth.	Full: Thyroid enlargement, perchlorate discharge.
	Partial: Low frequency[44]	Partial: Some of findings present perchlorate discharge, goiter at birth or 2nd decade. Mondini dysplasia common.

(continued)

Table 2–5. (continued)

Cause of Hearing Loss	Audiologic Signs	Other Characteristics
Integumentary		
Waardenburg syndrome	Variance bilateral; usually moderate severe; pan cochlear, Type II with frequent SNHL	Type I (dystopia canthorum) Type II (no dystopia canthorum)
Cardio-Vascular		
Jervell & Lange-Nielsen syndrome	Profound	Syncope at age 3–5, ECG: Prolonged QT interval
Skeletal Disease		
Treacher Collins syndrome	Conductive or mixed.	External auditory canal atresia,
Pierre Robin syndrome		Middle ear anomalies
Apert's syndrome	Variance of pure conductive and mixed; typically progressive	Premature; craniofacial synostosis-syndactyly
Crouzon's syndrome	"	Premature craniofacial synostosis
Klippel-Feil syndrome	"	Incidence Mondini dysplasia and ankylosed ossicles
Goldenhar syndrome	"	Klippel-Feil with preauricular appendages, low-set auricles
Wildervanck syndrome	"	Klippel-Feil with 6th Nerve palsy, external ear defect
Osteopetrosis (Albers Schönberg disease)	Progressive mixed conductive in low frequencies, SNHL in high at onset.	Onset in childhood, progression to deafness and blindness
Van Buchem syndrome		
Pyle syndrome		

Marfan syndrome, Paget's disease and van der Höeve syndrome are typically mixed hearing loss with onset early adult.

DIAGNOSTIC EXAMINATION AFTER IDENTIFICATION OF HEARING LOSS[45]

The following diagnostic approach is based on two fundamental considerations: (1) the major causes of bilateral SNHL (hereditary, viral, and so forth), and (2) the pediatric age groups in which physical and laboratory signs may become manifest. For example, the eye lesion in RP may not appear until age 6 years, but the hearing loss associated with this condition may be manifested much earlier.

Birth to 3 Years

Birth to 6 Months

In addition to the following procedures, blood agglutination and urine culture (mother and patient) should be done for CMV in the age group of birth to 3 years. If both are positive, this may be a presumptive cause of deafness.

1. CT scan for abnormal structure of cochlea, vestibular system, and internal auditory canals.
2. Urinalysis to rule out Alport's syndrome or other forms of kidney disease. More than three red blood cells (RBC) or five white cells (WBC) per high-powered field (HPF) or presence of protein is considered abnormal. This test should be followed by determinations of serum creatinine and blood urea nitrogen (BUN). Alport's syndrome should be considered with a SNHL of recent onset, regardless of the child's sex. Kidney manifestations that occur in infancy ("red diaper" syndrome), but hearing loss is not present until 8 to 10 years of age.
3. Urinalysis for mucopolysaccharidosis (MPS) prior to age 18 months. By 18 months, typical facies have formed and MPS can be suspected by physical examination. Be wary of false-positives. Confirmation of MPS should be made with blood agglutination or skin biopsy, or both. Although the condition is rare, the Sanfilippo syndrome does occur, but children will not show characteristics of the MPS until 4 to 5 years of age.
4. Vestibular examination.

Ages 3 to 6 Years

1. CT scan of temporal bone structures (if not done previously).
2. Ophthalmological examination for myopia or RP. RP cannot be diagnosed before age 3 unless it is congenital (a rare entity); between ages

3 and 6 it may or may not be diagnosed; and at age 6, it can definitely be diagnosed. Electroretinography (ERG) may permit the diagnosis in the presymptomatic state.
3. Electrocardiography (ECG) if patient has drop attacks, as in Jervell and Lange-Nielsen syndrome.
4. FTA-ABS for syphilis if there is onset of hearing loss in low frequencies.
5. Urinalysis for protein and blood cells.
6. Thyroxine (T_4) uptake or perchlorate discharge test if goiter is found or if history indicates.

Ages 6 to 9+ Years

1. Urinalysis for protein and blood cells.
2. FTA-ABS for syphilis if there is onset of hearing loss in low frequencies.
3. CT scan and EEG since neurological syndromes start to appear at age 8.

These tests have been found to be most efficacious in determining hearing loss on the basis of 127 children with SNHL.[45] Other tests, such as the perchlorate (if a thyroid goiter is found), a skull x-ray series (if osteopetrosis or other bony defects are suspected), and karyotype for cytogenetic disorders are done if indicated.

A CT scan is of no value in the early age groups, even when brain damage accompanies hearing loss. In those rare cases of unusual neurological signs, CT scans or EEGs are of little diagnostic value prior to either the first appearance of a bilateral hearing impairment or the associated complex of signs usually indicative of such hearing losses. These syndromes include those presenting with ataxia, which may appear when the child is 8 years of age or older.

To order all standard pediatric tests for assessing possible bilateral SNHL is self-defeating. Not only are such clinical tests an expensive use of medical resources, but their diagnostic projections are also very poor. When a 3-year-old child is identified as having a bilateral sensorineural hearing impairment, for example, there is no definitive confirmation that the auditory loss was caused by a CMV agent present at birth unless the appropriate viral screening studies were done during the neonatal period or shortly thereafter. Even when all possible causes other than viral are eliminated, the particular child may have come into contact with many different viruses during his or her first 3 years of life. Therefore, viral studies done at the age of 3 would be diagnostically superfluous. Such considerations have prompted a more systematic approach to diagnostic evaluation of bilateral SNHL in pediatric patients.

Hereditary hearing loss occurs with no associated abnormalities in about two thirds of patients. In the remaining one third, the loss is part of an identifiable syndrome of abnormalities. For some diagnoses, laboratory tests are needed for confirmation. The absence of findings (such as a lack of family history of hearing impairment) in hereditary hearing loss associated with no other abnormalities confirms no diagnosis. In such a family, the only confirmation of hereditary hearing loss would be existence of a second sibling with a similar defect.

The diagnosis of some syndromes cannot be confirmed or supported by laboratory data. A more common example (1 to 2% of all cases of congenital hearing loss)[46] is the diagnosis of Waardenburg syndrome, which has to be made by observation of the characteristic features in the patient or the family. Features of this syndrome vary, but most commonly include (1) lateral placement of the internal canthi and lacrimal punctum; (2) a prominent broad nasal root; (3) hypertrichosis of the eyebrows; (4) white forelock; (5) heterochromia of the irises; and (6) less common in occurrence, moderate to profound SNHL.[46]

It has been this author's experience that radiographic study of the inner ear has proved to be the most productive test in investigating SNHL. Inner ear structural defects, demonstrated by CT scan, were consistently the most common findings in a small group of children with SNHL enrolled in the Pappas ECHO* Foundation, Birmingham, Alabama, who had no other pathological manifestations.

MEDICAL MONITORING

There are cases in which a specific diagnosis cannot be confirmed (30%, author's statistics). The cause may emerge later in some of these cases. For example, the birth of a second offspring with SNHL would indicate inheritance, certain retinal changes would indicate RP, changes in other organs may become recognized and a syndrome identified, or a family may cease to be reticent about history.[47]

Although audiometric evaluation in SNHL is frequently recommended according to needs, evaluations for etiology should be repeated at least every 3 years. Even those patients in whom the cause has been determined should be reexamined to confirm the diagnosis.

*ECHO is an acronym for Equilibrium-Communication-Hearing-Otology.

DEVELOPMENTAL
SPEECH-LANGUAGE
SCREENING

Children with severe to profound SNHL are very difficult to test with developmental screening tests, since typically without amplification there is no verbal development in the early years. One should add, however, an assessment of language development, such as the Early Language Milestone Scale[48] for all patients (normal hearing and mild to moderate hearing losses). It is helpful in detecting language delay from various causes, and only adds a minute or two to the examination.

POSTDIAGNOSIS
IMPLEMENTATIONS

The physician's role goes beyond the restoration of hearing to as near normal levels as possible. His or her responsibility also encompasses the prevention and correction of speech and language disorders that may accompany the hearing loss, including the determination and remediation of any associated learning disabilities. For those children in whom a hearing loss is suspected, remediation should be instituted immediately. Amplification in infants with conductive hearing loss may precede surgery, as in patients with bilateral external auditory atresia. Speech and language development should be observed closely, and special education should be provided as indicated. Progress in communication skills and educational development must be monitored every 6 months, and any changes in habilitation therapy should be instituted as soon as possible.

In those cases in which anomalies and hearing loss are common, such as cleft palate and middle ear effusions, immediate surgical intervention with ventilation tubes is a prudent course of action.

Above all, the physician must be aware of the social, psychological, and educational consequences of speech and language delays that may result from a sensorineural or conductive hearing loss. The medical rehabilitation and educational success of any child hearing-impaired depend on early diagnosis and appropriate treatment. Bilateral SNHL is all too frequently overlooked in infancy and early childhood; it becomes "invisible" through incomplete medical histories and inadequate physical examinations. The physician's role in the early identification of SNHL in a child is, indeed, critical.

SUMMARY

Abnormalities associated with hearing loss are listed in this chapter. It has been the experience of the author that, when true syndromes are present and obvious, the constellation of findings have been identified by the pediatrician and geneticist. The patient is then referred for otological findings, especially for a hearing evaluation. Typically, those initially seen by the otolaryngologist have no physical findings or at best, subtle findings.

In performing this type of work, the physician must have "fingertip" knowledge or information and be able to synthesize the information to form a diagnosis. For example, syphilis does not cause hearing loss in infancy (usually hearing loss caused by syphilis emerges at age 8), the syncope of Jervill and Lange-Nielsen syndrome does not show until age 3-5; Alport's deafness at age 8, and so on.

REFERENCES

1. Schuknecht HF. Mondini dysplasia-a clinical and pathological study. *Ann Otol Rhinol Laryngol*. 1980;89(suppl 65):3-23.
2. Pappas DG, Simpson LC, Godwin GH. Perilymphatic fistula in children with preexisting sensorineural hearing loss, *Laryngoscope*. 1988;98:507-510.
3. Rosenhall U, Kankkunen A. Hearing alterations following meningitis. Variable hearing. *Ear Hear*. 1981;2:170-178.
4. Brookhouser PE. Early recognition of childhood hearing impairment. *J Ear Nose Throat*. 1979;58:19.
5. Blakely RW. Erythroblastosis and perceptive hearing loss: responses of athetoids to tests of cochlear function. *J Speech Hear Res*. 1959;2:5-15.
6. Vernon M. Prematurity and deafness: the magnitude and nature of the problem among deaf children. *Except Child*. 1967;33:289-298.
7. Vernon M. Rh factor and deafness. *Except Child*. 1967; 34:5-12.
8. Bordley JE, Hardy JM. Laboratory and clinical observations on prenatal rubella. *Ann Otol Ehinol Laryngol*. 1969;78:917-927.
9. Johnsson L-G, Hawkins JE Jr. Symposium on basic ear research. II. Strial atrophy in clinical and experimental deafness. *Laryngoscope*. 1972;82:1105-1125.
10. Hawkins JE Jr. Ototoxic mechanisms: a working hypothesis. *Audiology*. 1973;12:383-393.
11. Myers EN, Bernstein JM, Fostiropolous G. Salicylate ototoxicity. *N Engl J Med*. 1965;273:587-590.
12. McCabe PA, Dey FL. The effect of aspirin upon auditory sensitivity. *Ann Otol*. 1965;74:313-325.
13. Hennebert D, Fernandez C. Ototoxicity of quinine in experimental animals. *Arch Otolaryngol*. 1959;70:321-333.

14. McKinna AJ. Quinine induced hypoplasia of the optic nerve. *Can J Ophthalmol.* 1966;1:261-266.
15. Hart CW, Naunton RF. The ototoxicity of chloroquine phosphate. *Arch Otolaryngol.* 1964;80:407-411.
16. Matz GJ, Naunton RF. Ototoxicity of chloroquine. *Arch Otolaryngol.* 1968;88:370-72.
17. Keleman G. Maternal diabetes. Changes in the hearing organ of the embryo: Additional observation. *Arch Otolaryngol.* 1960;71:921-925.
18. Jorgensen MB. Influence of maternal diabetes on the inner ear of the foetus. *Acta Otolaryngol.* 1960;53:49-54.
19. American Academy Joint Committee on Infant Hearing 1990 Position Statement. AAO-HNS Bulletin March 1991.
20. Feingold M. Clinical evaluation of a patient with a genetic or birth defect syndrome. *Am J Med Sci.* 1982;19:151-156.
21. Pappas DG, Schaibly M. A two-year diagnostic report on bilateral sensorineural hearing loss in infants and children. *Am J Otol.* 1984;5:339-343.
22. Stagno S, Pass RF, Alford CA. Perinatal infections and maldevelopment. *Birth Defects.* 1981;17:31-50.
23. Paparella MM, Goycoolea MV, Meyerhoff WL. Inner ear pathology and otitis media: a review. In: Recent advances in otitis media with effusion. *Ann Otol Rhinol Laryngol.* 1980;89(suppl 68):249-253.
24. Caldarelli DD. Congenital middle ear anomalies associated with craniofacial and skeletal syndromes. In: Jaffe BF, ed. *Hearing Loss in Children.* Baltimore, Md: University Park Press; 1977:301-314.
25. Dunn PM. Congenital postural deformities. *Br Med Bull.* 1976;32:71-76.
26. Marden PM, Smith DW, McDonald MJ. Congenital anomalies in the newborn infant, including minor variations. *J Pediatr.* 1964;64:371-375.
27. Feingold M. Clinical evaluation of a patient with a genetic or birth defect syndrome. *Alabama J Med Sci.* 1982;19:151-156.
28. Jaffe BF. Middle ear and pinna anomalies. In: Jaffe BF. *Hearing Loss in Children.* Baltimore, Md: University Press; 1977:294-309.
29. Altmann F. Congenital atresia of the ear in man and animals. *Ann Rhinol Laryngol.* 1955;64:824-857.
30. Naunton RF, Valvassori GE. Inner ear anomalies: their association with atresia. *Laryngoscope.* 1968;78:1041-1049.
31. Doyle WJ, Cantekin EI, Bluestone CD. Eustachian tube function in cleft palate children. In: Recent advances in otitis media with effusion. *Ann Otol Rhinol Laryngol.* 1980; 89(suppl 68):34-40.
32. Konigsmark BW, Gorlin RJ. *Genetic and Metabolic Deafness.* Philadelphia, Pa: WB Saunders; 1976:74-134.
33. Fisch L. Deafness as part of an hereditary syndrome. *J Laryngol Otol.* 1959: 73:355 382.
34. Enbom H, Magnusson M, Pyykko I. Postural compensation in children with congenital or early acquired bilateral hearing loss. *Otol. Rhinol. Laryngol.* 1991;100:472-478.

35. Oliveira C, Schuknecht H. Pathology of profound sensorineural hearing loss in infancy and early childhood. *Laryngoscope.* August 1990;100:902-909.
36. Bárány R. Untersuchungen über den vom vestibularapparat des ohres reflektorisch ausgelösten rhythmischen nystagmus und seine begleiterscheinungen. In: *Monatschrift für Ohrenheilkunde,* [Researches in the rhythmic nystagmus reflected from the vestibular apparatus of the ear and its accompanying symptoms],1906;40:193-297.
37. Wolfe JW, Engelken EJ, Kos CM. Low-frequency harmonic acceleration as a test of labyrinthine function: basic methods and illustrative cases. *Trans Am Acad Ophthalmol Otorlaryngol.* 1978;86:130-142.
38. Wolfe JW, Engelken EJ, Olson, JW, Kos CM. Vestibular responses to bithermal caloric and harmonic acceleration. *Ann Otol Rhinol Laryngol.* 1978;87:861-867.
39. Wolfe JW, Kos CM. Nystagmic responses of the Rhesus monkey to rotational stimulation following unilateral labyrinthectomy: final report. *Trans Am Acad Ophthalmol Otolaryngol.* 1977;84:38-45.
40. Wolfe JW, Engelken EJ, Olson E. Low frequency harmonic acceleration in evaluation of patients with peripheral labyrinthine disorders. In: Honrubia V, ed. *Nystagmus and Vertigo: Clinical Approaches to the Patient with Dizziness.* New York, NY: Academic Press; 1982.
41. Fernandez C, Goldberg JM. Physiology of the peripheral neurons innervating semicircular canals of the squirrel monkey. II. Response to sinusoidal stimulation and dynamics of peripheral vestibular system. *J Neurophysiol.* 1971; 34:661-675.
42. Baloh RW, Honruhia JV , Konrad HR. Ewald's second law reevaluated. *Acta Otolaryngol.* 1977;83:475-479.
43. Wilson VJ, Jones MG. *Mammalian Vestibular Physiology.* New York, NY: Plenum Press; 1979:53.
44. Jamal MN, Arnaout MA, Jarrar R, Jordan A. Penred's Syndrome: a study of patients and relatives. *Ann otol Rhinol Laryngol.* December 1995:104(12): 957-962.
45. Pappas DG, Mundy MR: Sensorineural hearing loss in young children: a systematic approach to evaluation. *South Med J.* 1981;74:965-967.
46. Fraser GR. *The Causes of Profound Deafness in Childhood.* Baltimore, Md: Johns Hopkins University Press; 1976.
47. Pappas DG. A study of the high-risk registry for sensorineural hearing impairment. *Otolaryngol Head Neck Surg.* 1983;91:41-44.
48. Coplan J. *The Early Language Milestone Scale.* Tulsa, Ok, Modern Education Corporation, 1983.

CHAPTER

3

Fundamentals of Inheritance

A study of family portraits is enough to convert a man to the doctrine of reincarnation.
The Hound of the Baskervilles
Sherlock Holmes

I have frequently gained my first real insight into the character of parents by studying their children.
The Adventure of Copper Beeches
Sherlock Holmes

During the time infectious diseases such as smallpox, cholera, and diphtheria were rampant, an Austrian botanist and monk, Gregor Johann Mendel (1822-1884), discovered the principles of genetic transmission.

His experiments in growing garden peas demonstrated that selective breeding made it possible to produce peas displaying ratios of characters that permitted the recognition of a recessive or a dominant trait. However, because of the lack of a significant correlation between inheritance and disease, the application of genetic transmission to clinical medicine developed slowly. Early genetic studies were concerned with the preservation of life and improvement of human conditions. As recently as the 1920s, scarlet fever ravaged the kidneys, heart, joints, and hearing because doctors could offer only empirical treatment. Therefore, such problems as infectious diseases, with their potentially devastating effects on both adults and children, took precedence over research into the transmission of genetic traits. The chain of events in medical genetics and the scientists behind them is a fascinating one and is outlined in Table 3–1.

Table 3–1. Important Dates in Medical Genetics*

BC		
	1000	Babylonians—Religious ritual, pollination of date palm tree
	323	Aristotle—inheritance
	100–300	Indian writings on human reproduction
AD		
	1676	Grew—sex in plants
	1677	Leeuwenhoek—saw animal sperm
	1716	Mather—cross-pollination in maize
	1838	Living organisms composed of cells
	1859	Darwin—Origin of Species
	1865	Mendel—gave paper on peas
	1866	Mendel published paper
	1868	Darwin—variations in animals and plants
	1871	Miescher—"nuclein"
	1875	Hertwig—fertilization of sea-urchin egg
	1882–1885	Chromosome behavior worked out in some detail
	1883	Roux—mitosis
	1883	Galton coined eugenics
	1883–1889	Weismann—germ-plasm theory
	1889	Altmann—nucleic acid
	1894	Bateson—study of variation
	1900	Correns, De Vries, Tschermak—rediscovery of Mendel
	1900	Landsteiner—human blood groups
	1901	McClung—X chromosome
	1901	De Vries—Die mutations Theorie

1902	Bateson & Cuenot—Mendelism in animals
1902	Boveri—individuality of the chromosomes
1902	Correns—time and place of segregation
1903	Levine—chemical distinction between DNA & ANA
1903	Sutton—chromosomes and Mendelism
1904	Cuenot —multiple alleles
1905	Bateson & Punnett—linkage
1905	Stevens & Wilson—sex chromosomes and sex determination
1906	Doncaster & Raynor—sex linkage
1907	Marchal & Lutz—polyploidy
1908	Garrod—alkaptonuria
1908	Hardy-Weinberg equilibrium
1908	Lutz—trisomy
1908	Nilsson-Ehle—multiple gene interpretation
1909	Correns—plastid inheritance
1909	Janssens—chiasma
1909	Johannsen—Elemente der exakte Erblichkeitslehre
1909	Johannsen —coined gene
1914	Boveri—disturbance in chromosome balance
1927	Muller—x-rays cause mutations
1944	Avery et al—DNA was genetic material
1949	Barr & Bertram —discovered X chromatin
1949	Pauling et al—sickle cell anemia due to abnormal hemogoblin
1953	Watson, Crick—DNA model
1956	Levan & Tjio—chromosome no. of man
1959	Lejeune—discovered 21 trisomy in DS
1960	Patau described trisomy 13; Edwards trisomy 18
1960	Nowell, Hungerford—described Ph' chromosome in CML
1960	Moorhead—chromosome preparations from leucocytes
1961	Jacob, Monod—unit of gene action (operon)
1961	Nirenberg, Matthael—triplet code
1963	Lejeune—described Cri-du-Chat 5p syndrome
1970	Caspersson—chromosome banding techniques

*Presented to the author by Wayne Finley, MD, University of Alabama, Birmingham.

The introduction of antibiotics in the 1940s greatly alleviated the threats to life associated with many illnesses, and the intensive research into genetics began. In the 1950s, methods were devised to accurately study chromosomes, and for the first time the actual number of chromosomes in the normal human (46, or 22 pairs of autosomal chromosomes and one pair of sex chromosomes) became known. Soon a number of various abnormalities in number and structure were identified, some of which were associated with an increase in the total number of chromosomes. One of the most common of these is the occurrence of an extra chromosome 21.

The study of chromosomes has now been refined to the point that the individual portions of the chromosomes can be identified. This progress allows the accurate description of chromosomal aberrations and, consequently, more accurate genetic counseling and management. Chromosome studies can be carried out in a variety of clinical situations. This field (human cytogenetics) has made tremendous progress since the 1950s and has passed through three phrases. The first, starting in 1956 and continuing into the late 1960s, was that of chromosome analysis that detected abnormalities of chromosome number and a few structural aberrations. Conditions discovered during this time were, for example, the trisomies 13, 18, and 21. The second stage of progression, occurring in the 1970s, was that of the introduction of banning techniques that led to the discovery of a large number of interstitial and terminal deletions and duplications (eg, mosaic tetrasomy 12P syndrome). The third stage, introduced in the 1980s, was the development of methods for identifying microdeletions and for gene mapping (microdeletion syndromes) (ie, Prader-Willi syndrome). Typically, chromosome studies should be done on all patients with a suspected chromosome syndrome to confirm the diagnosis, or in any patient with multiple malformations when the overall diagnosis is unknown.[1]

Clinically, such cases present with hearing loss in the following manner: conductive, SNHL, mixed, or any of the preceding associated with syndromes. Inability to decipher the intricate embryological interaction of thousands of cells making up the inner, middle, and outer ear is compounded by the lack of knowledge concerning normal fetal development, much less abnormal development. It is known, however, that hereditary factors are present in many cases of infertility, miscarriages, neonatal deaths, multiple malformations, growth disturbances, mental retardation, and some mental illnesses.[2]

MAGNITUDE OF THE PROBLEM

Each year between 2000 and 4000 infants who are profoundly hearing-impaired are born in the United States[3], and of these, approximately 30 to 50%[4] of cases may be classified as genetically based, and probably over one third are syndromal (that is, associated with other anomalies). These figures indicate that hereditary deafness is not rare.

Twenty-five percent of congenital hearing loss is of the acquired type and in 30% of the children evaluated, the hearing loss is of undetermined etiology. One in 1000 children in the well-born nursery will have deafness of a degree significant enough to interfere with speech and language development. In the intensive care nursery 1 to 2 out of 50 infants have appreciable hearing loss. These figures are checked by us every year in our own clinical practice and tend to be consistent over the last several decades. According to Gorlin et al, there are 23 types of hereditary hearing loss with no associated abnormalities identified at this time.[1]

Another problem is that of financial remuneration of those who are hearing-impaired. The people who are deaf earn 30% less than the typically hearing population. In addition, there are 21 million people with lesser degrees of hearing loss who have income decrement as a result. As one compares those with congenital deafness with those who have had normal hearing until age 3, there is a 5% improvement in income.[5] Thus, if hearing impairment is detected at birth and intervention occurs early, there could be the possibility of reducing the cost to society associated with hearing-impairment.[6] Obviously, school performance has been well-documented to correlate with job performance and financial rewards later in life.

HISTORY TAKING FOR INHERITANCE

The parents of a child with an inherited hearing loss certainly have a greater risk of having other children with hearing impairment. The implications of this make it imperative that the diagnosis of inherited deafness be correct. It has been shown that the hearing loss in a significant number of children who have been classified as having an inherited hearing defect actually could have resulted from a subclinical viral infection.[7] As the child matures, laboratory testing cannot determine if the hearing loss is caused by hereditary factors or is the result of a viral infection. Of course, if a viral cause could be determined, it would eliminate genetic implications.

Hereditary hearing loss must be identified on the basis of a thorough medical and family history, which should include the following:

1. Determination of the cause and circumstances under which the hearing impairment was first noticed. The term "deafness" includes a group of distinct pathological conditions that may be caused by any one of, or a combination of, various factors and agents. For instance, the damage to the auditory pathways caused by the rubella virus was acquired in the prenatal period. Thus, this condition is acquired, but congenital,[8] since the condition occurred at or before birth. On the other hand, hereditary hearing loss is congenital when the hearing loss is present at birth, but it is hereditary as well as congenital. When hearing is normal at birth and the loss is manifested only some years later and

causes for an acquired loss have been ruled out, the condition is considered delayed hereditary. In other words, not all cases of genetic hearing impairment are necessarily congenital. An example of this mistaken assumption is Alport's syndrome, in which the hearing loss tends to appear at 8 years of age.

As suggested in Chapter 2 and outlined in Table 2–3 of that chapter, use of the term "delayed" may allow the term "acquired" to be reserved for those cases of postpartum deafness resulting from extrinsic causes. In any case, the purpose of classifications and differential diagnosis is to facilitate early identification, habilitation, and prognosis for progression of the hearing loss.

2. A complete family history, including a history of all of the mother's pregnancies (prior and subsequent to the patient's birth).
3. An additional family history of genetic data relating to the patient's extended and immediate family members (especially any indication of hearing impairment or learning difficulties among the relatives).
4. A thorough, complete (total body) physical examination, with particular inspection of the head and neck regions to detect obvious malformations. Hereditary hearing impairment may accompany disorders of other systems.
5. Selective testing procedures for assessing possible causes of SNHL (see Chapter 2).

Despite all of the progress that has been made in psychogenetics, it is still very difficult to differentiate a hearing loss of inheritance from one of viral origin. Important features to consider, in the working diagnosis are:

1. Dominant features.
2. Second or more siblings with SNHL.
3. Consanguinity.
4. Features of twins.

A more detailed outline of the current criteria for diagnosing genetic diseases may be found elsewhere.[9]

TYPES OF DISORDERS OR ALTERATIONS IN GENETIC MATERIALS

In sexually reproducing organisms, the normal mechanisms of inheritance follow a precise trail that begins with the events of meiosis and ends with fertilization and the development of a new offspring. This pathway leads the predictable transmission of chromosomes, genes, and genetic traits between generations.

Occasionally, however, deviations in normal genetic processes lead to abnormal combinations or a modification in the structure of genes or chromosomes within the cells. A permanent structural change within the hereditary material is called a mutation. The end result of a mutation— the effect on the offspring—can vary dramatically: there may be no effect, new variants (offspring with new forms of a trait) may appear, or premature death may occur before or after birth. In the transmission of characteristics from parent to offspring, three major groups of genetic disease affect humans: (1) Mendelian disorders caused by a single gene (autosomal dominant, autosomal recessive, X-linked inheritance), (2) cytogenetic disorders (chromosomal aberrations), and (3) multifactorial genetic diseases (Table 3–2). A fresh mutation, resulting in a change either in the gene or in the somatic cells, is not a common cause of genetic transmission of traits.[10]

Normally, every person inherits two genes (the units of heredity, formed of coded information) for a particular trait, one from the mother and one from the father. Hundreds of genes, arranged in a line, are carried on the length of each chromosome. The physical traits of the individual are determined by the pattern these genes assume and their clinical expression. Because of gene-gene interaction and environmental effects, the same gene in two individuals may have different manifestations.

Patterns of Inheritance

Autosomal Dominant

Genes may be described as dominant or recessive. Those that express their effect when present in only a single "dose" are known as dominant genes; these appear in successive generations. Autosomal dominant inheritance is responsible for 20 to 25% of hereditary hearing impairment.[11] There is a probability that any child of a parent with a dominant hearing disorder will also have that disorder. Although one of the characteristics of Mendelian dominant inheritance (equal numbers in equal proportions) will be present, expression of the trait varies in degree among those who are affected. Thus, the hearing loss may be unilateral or bilateral.[12] At times, the abnormal gene fails to show dominance altogether; this is known as failure of penetrance of the affected gene, and there is no detectable expression of its characteristics. This phenomenon is seen with dominantly inherited disorders in which the grandmother has the condition, the father does not, and the grandson does. There is no

Table 3–2. Patterns of Inherited Disorders

Single Gene

Autosomal dominant disorders

Autosomal recessive disorders

X-linked disorders

Cytogenetic and Chromosomal Abnormalities

Trisomy syndromes (Duplication or increase in amount of genetic material)	**Sex chromosome syndromes**
Down's	Turner's syndrome (XO)
Trisomy 18	Klinefelter's syndrome (XXY)
Trisomy 13–15	XYY syndrome
	X-linked mental retardation

Deletion syndromes (Loss of a segment chromosome)	**Chromosome instability (Inversions, shifts, of translocations)**
	Xeroderma pigmentosum
4p	Bloom's syndrome
Cri-du-chat (5p)	Fanconi's anemia
13q	Ataxia-telangiectasia
18q	Prader-Willi Syndrome

Multifactorial or Polygenic Inheritance

Single or multiple gene defect with environmental factors.

Example: Cleft lip/palate.

Features:

1. Reoccurrence in relatives greater than that of general population.
2. Chance of trait increases with each additional family member affected.
3. The more severe the malformation, the greater the risk to relatives.

Modified with permission from Gorlin et al.[1]

expression of the gene in the second generation or, perhaps, the expression is so mild that it is unidentifiable by available methods.[13]

Autosomal dominant hearing disorders also vary in severity ("variable expressivity"), and progression of hearing loss is common in many of these cases. The author has seen a patient with Waardenburg's syndrome and severe to profound, bilateral SNHL who, earlier in life, had had a flat audiometric configuration that progressed to a "corner audiogram." Typically, patients with dominantly inherited hearing loss will have flat, moderate to severe audiometric threshold levels. Some, however, show a high frequency hearing loss. Therefore, classification of the type or cause of the hearing impairment should not be attempted on the basis of audiometric patterns alone.

Autosomal Recessive

Autosomal recessive inheritance accounts for 75 to 80% of the cases of hereditary hearing impairment.[11] Recessive genes are those that are expressed only when a "double dose" is present; that is, the child gets the same abnormal (or normal) gene from each parent. In the case of deafness, the clinical manifestation of a pair of recessive genes in an offspring depends on the presence of the gene in both parents, who have two unlike genes (normally in pairs), one normal and one abnormal (heterozygote), at the same chromosome locus. In other words, an abnormal gene from each parent is required for expression of this type of hearing impairment. An example of recessive transmission is Usher's syndrome.

It is estimated that one person in eight is a carrier of a recessive form of hearing impairment.[14] Because there are so many different types of recessive hearing loss, the probability of matching the specific abnormal gene is low, and the risk of having a child who is hearing-impaired is decreased. The chances of having a child with a hearing loss as a consequence of the linkage of two identically abnormal genes (one from each parent) is 25%. The parents of a child with a recessive inheritance form of hearing impairment are usually normal. Autosomal recessive hearing losses tend to be symmetrical and more severe than those of autosomal dominant inheritance, although audiometric patterns vary. Many infants with "corner audiograms" have recessive hearing impairment, probably reflecting the fact that most cases of recessive hearing loss are associated with the Scheibe deformity of the cochlea, and predominantly affect the organ of Corti, stria vascularis, and tectorial membrane.

There is an increased incidence of recessive inheritance found in marriages with common ancestry (such as a marriage of cousins). This type of union increases the possibility that each parent will be a carrier of the identical defective gene that may express itself as an abnormal trait in their child.

X-Linked

This type of inheritance pattern became known primarily because of its role in the transmission of hemophilia in the royal families of Europe. Color blindness is also an X-linked trait. X-linked recessive hearing losses form a smaller number of congenital cases (up to 3%).[11]

Each male individual has, in addition to his 22 pairs of autosomal chromosomes, two sex chromosomes, X and Y; the latter chromosome determines that the individual is a male. The female has two X chromosomes. In X-linked recessive traits, the genes for SNHL are located on the X chromosome and can occur in both dominant and recessive forms, although most are thought to react in a recessive fashion. The risk that an X-linked recessive trait will be transmitted from a carrier mother to any of her sons is 50%. Consequently, when the son has an X-linked recessive defect, he must have derived the X chromosome carrying the abnormal gene from his mother, since there can be no father-to-son transmission of an X-linked recessive trait (sons receive only the Y chromosome from their fathers). A carrier female with a single abnormal X-linked recessive gene could have affected or normal sons; her daughters or the mother herself may manifest the disorder in a modified form, such as a mild SNHL. With the exception of a rare group characterized by fixation of the footplate,[15] X-linked recessive hearing losses are sensorineural, and frequently there is some retention of hearing in all frequencies.

CYTOGENETIC DISORDERS

Cytogenetic disorders are caused either by errors in the distribution of the chromosomes or by structural changes in one or more of the chromosomes. Down's syndrome, the most autosomal aberration syndrome,[16] occurs in one of every 600 to 800 live births and is usually the result of an extra chromosome 21 (Fig 3–1, A). Approximately 5% of Down's syndrome cases are due to the translocation and fusion of part of chromosome 21 to chromosome 14. Cytogenetic analysis is indicated in patients with cytogenic disorders to define the precise nature of the abnormality and allow appropriate genetic counseling for the family. One method of cytogenetic analysis is the karyotype technique, for which only a small sample of heparinized blood is needed. By special processing, including leukocyte culture, arresting cells at metaphase, and arranging the chromosomes of a single cell in pairs, a karyotype is constructed[16] (Fig 3–2).

Down's Syndrome

One of the most frequently observed clinical conditions associated with mental retardation is Down's syndrome. During the first few years of life, a large percentage of these children are only mildly or moderately retarded and, indeed, some appear to be of average intelligence. However, a subsequent decline in measured intelligence is well-documented.[17] The

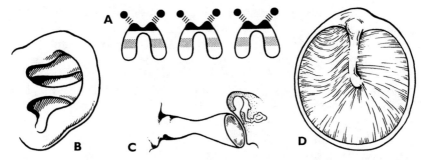

Fig 3-1.—Features of Down's syndrome. A, Trisomy pattern of chromosome 21. B, Small concha that may be typical in children with Down's syndrome. C, "Hourglass" stenosis of external auditory canal. D, Schematic illustration of early retraction of posterior-inferior portion of tympanic membrane caused by chronic eustachian tube obstruction.

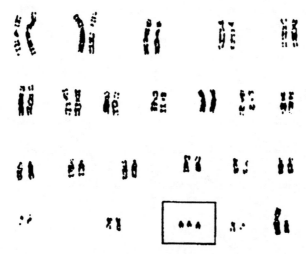

Fig 3-2.—Karyotype typical of Down's syndrome.

impact of certain health-related problems (especially otological) on the development of intelligence is still obscure.[18] It has been shown, however, that children with Down's syndrome, when compared with other children with and without retardation of the same mental age, are delayed in their development.[19,20] Specifically, these children show widely variable learning characteristics, especially in the acquisition of traditional verbal instructions.[21] Otological problems possibly contribute to this delay in development.

The relatively high incidence of hearing loss in the population with Down's syndrome is well-documented.[22-24] In children with this syndrome, three factors may hinder hearing performance during the early years: (1) the high incidence of stenosis of the external auditory canal, (2) the high incidence of serous otitis media (SOM), and (3) the increased incidence of cholesteatoma or keratoma. These characteristic otological findings in children with Down's syndrome, apparently not shared by other children who are mentally retarded, may further hamper their acquisition of language skills. The stenotic auditory canal of children with Down's syndrome has the appearance of an hourglass with the narrowed segment located at the junction of the cartilaginous and bony portions of the canal (Fig 3–1, C). The stenosis is composed of a soft tissue thickening and is not usually a bony narrowing. Older children with Down's syndrome do not have such small ear canals, which may indicate that the thickened canal tissue recedes and forms a more normal-sized external auditory canal. However, in some the canal is stenotic in the formative years of speech and language development (birth to 3 years of age). This stenosis may vary, and in some cases the canal is so narrow that even small specks of cerumen can block the canal and the air conduction pathways of hearing. Moreover, such a configuration of the canal may make visualization of the eardrum impossible. The inability to visualize the eardrum and the typical cheerful, pleasant, and uncomplaining personality of children with Down's syndrome, make them unusually susceptible to an undiagnosed chronic SOM that may later produce a retraction cholesteatoma (Fig 3–1, D).

Conductive hearing loss associated with Down's syndrome varies from 15 to 40 dB above normal threshold and is usually associated with the factors mentioned in the previous paragraph. Balkany and coworkers reported that SNHL was encountered in approximately 17% of their patients with Down's syndrome.[24] The degree of hearing loss varies in intensity, but it is rarely profound. Pathohistological studies revealed the cochlea to be slightly shorter in children with Down's syndrome than in controls, although individual structures appeared normal.[25]

Monitoring for Otological Problems

Infants with Down's syndrome should be evaluated early for a SNHL (by age 3 months). Although severe-to-profound hearing loss is not common in this group of children, the incidence of mild-to-moderate SNHL is statistically significant enough to warrant early investigation, identification, and amplification with hearing aids. The possibility of SNHL in cases of Down's syndrome being acquired as a delayed type of hearing loss is not fully appreciated at this time.[26]

Amplification with bone conduction aids may be recommended for infants with conductive hearing losses caused by extreme stenosis of the external auditory canal. Air conduction hearing aids usually do not work well in these cases because the mold cannot be stabilized in the concha (Fig 3–1, B). After the early years of temporal bone growth, the external canal usually enlarges.

Patients with Down's syndrome, especially in their early years, should be checked every 3 months for the presence of cerumen. In most of these children, a "speck of wax" in the stenotic ear canal can impede air conduction hearing. Even after removal of any cerumen, only a small portion of the tympanic membrane may be visible through a stenotic canal. Therefore, after removing the cerumen, tympanometry should be employed to check for negative pressure or fluid in the middle ear. Prolonged negative middle ear pressure must be avoided as it may lead to complications such as cholesteatoma or symptoms manifested in localized areas of the tympanic membrane.

Implanting a ventilation tube through a stenotic ear canal is often a difficult task for the surgeon. The tube must have a small lumen and small external diameter (0.76 mm). Unfortunately, this smallness in diameter makes the tube susceptible to blockage from serous debris and to premature extrusion within 4 to 6 months.

There is data suggesting a relationship between Down's syndrome and SNHL, including the relatively high incidence of SNHL and other otological deficits in the child's first years of speech and language development; the proneness of children with the syndrome to develop middle ear fluid, resulting in hearing loss levels of 25 to 30 dB and superimposed on subnormal mental levels; and studies indicating auditory-verbal skills that are inferior to those of children with other mental deficiencies.[21] Early detection and treatment of otological problems in patients with Down's syndrome would undoubtedly result in their developing better communication skills and, possibly, a higher level of academic achievement. In a pilot study in which the author was involved, a comparison was made of the language development of six infants with Down's syndrome who received aggressive treatment during their first year of life to six infants who did not. The proposed intervention plan began in the first 6 months of life and continued throughout childhood. The study showed that the model had the potential of achieving its targeted objective. The strongest statement that can be made is that early intervention is critical for the development of oral expressive language skills. Therefore, physicians were advised to refer infants with Down's syndrome for comprehensive audiologic management and speech-language therapy in their first 6 months of life.[27]

Trisomy 13–15, 18

Trisomy, or the presence of an extra chromosome, has been associated with SNHL and malformations of the middle and external ear in addition to that found in Down's syndrome. The most common trisomies, other than 21, involve chromosomes 13–15 and 18. Some of the common ear anomalies found in patients with trisomies 13–15 and 18 include low-set ears, poorly differentiated pinna, preauricular tags, absence or stenosis of the external auditory canal, and absence of the middle ear. Microscopic findings are varied[28-31] and may include Scheibe dysplasia, Mondini dysplasia, widened cochlear aqueduct, and communicating scalae.

Multifactorial Form of Genetic Malformation

Certain defects occur that do not follow the traditional laws of genetics. According to McKusick,[13] multifactorial inheritance refers to a collaboration of multiple genetic and nongenetic environmental factors to produce a particular disorder. The rare examples in this group of defects include spina bifida and anencephaly. Cleft lip and cleft palate are more common in occurrence, although the specific environmental factors in these cases have not been identified. Indeed, cleft lip and cleft palate may be the result of more than one gene, perhaps in conjunction with an environmental factor. These malformations tend to recur within families, and the chances of recurrence in a family with an affected child are increased, but not as greatly as for Mendelian inheritance.

Additional evidence of possible genetic-environmental collaboration to produce disease may be seen in some infectious diseases and, perhaps, fetal alcohol syndrome. Using animal-human hybrid cells, it has been demonstrated that chromosomes 5 and 19 carry genetic determinants for cell surface receptors that permit diphtheria toxin and poliovirus to enter the cells.[13]

PATHOPHYSIOLOGY OF HEARING IMPAIRMENT

Congenital and Delayed Onset Hereditary Type

The histopathology of congenital and delayed SNHL can be divided into two groups: those in which the bony labyrinth is normal and the neuroepithelium (organ of Corti) is abnormal, and those in which the bony labyrinth is abnormal and the neuroepithelium may or may not be normal (bony or Mondini dysplasia).[32,33] The histological classifications of these types of inner ear malformations were determined at the turn of this century. Other dysplasias mentioned in the literature include those of Michel, Alexander, and Bing-Siebenmann and are rare or difficult to document clinically.

Membranous Dysplasias

The failure of the organ of Corti and its associated membranes to develop (Scheibe dysplasia) is one of the most commonly found abnormalities in the pathological studies of SNHL patients. Hearing impairment as a result of this type of dysplasia may be inherited or, less frequently, be acquired during fetal development as a result of a virus (rubella[34]) or a drug (chloroquine[35]).

Characteristics of Scheibe dysplasia include a rudimentary organ of Corti, sparse or missing hair cells, distorted and collapsed supporting cells (Fig 3–3, A,B). The vestibular membrane is usually collapsed, but the utricle and semicircular canals are histologically and functionally normal.[36] One study of cell kinetics of the inner ear showed that the organ of Corti is composed of end-stage cells[37]; that is, after the cells are formed, they are unable to reproduce themselves. This would result in a hearing loss at any time after the second month of intrauterine life since the cells of the organ of Corti are probably formed during this time. Other studies have provided evidence to support hereditary delayed development of hearing loss.[38-40] In these animals, hair cells were present, but degeneration occurred shortly before or after birth. Not all cases of congenital or delayed onset hereditary hearing loss are Scheibe dysplasias. In fact, there is variability in the expression of pathological findings. A discussion of these is not warranted without further evidence and additional histopathological studies. However, it is known that recessive disorders tend to be related to metabolic defects and dominant disorders are most commonly seen with defects of structural genes.[13]

Membranous defects such as those just described cannot be diagnosed clinically. They may only be assumed on the basis of historical information and x-ray findings of normal bony structures. However, descriptions of the pathological findings in the temporal bones with correlations to the hearing loss have given us more insight into these defects.

Labyrinth and Petrous Bone

Bony Dysplasias

Inner ear malformations may be of hereditary, syndromal, or isolated origin. Drugs (Thalidomide) and viruses[41] (although not fully confirmed) are causes of isolated inner ear malformations.

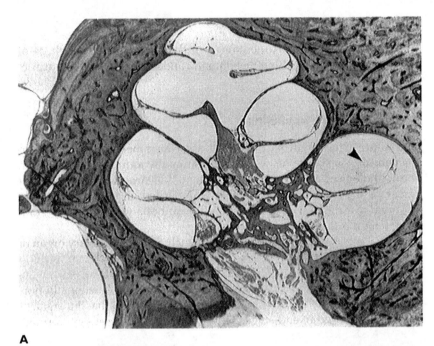

A

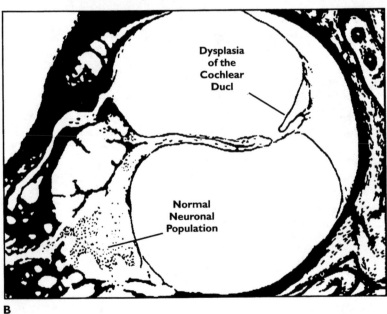

B

Fig 3-3.—A, Microscopic section of temporal bone in Scheibe dysplasia. Courtesy of Vincent Hyams, MD, Armed Forces Institute of Pathology, Washington, DC. B, Artist's rendering of the findings of the cochlear turn (arrowhead in A).

Cochlear malformations include Mondini dysplasia, aplasia, hypoplasia, and dilation.

Cochlear aplasia, where sclerotic bone is seen in place of the cochlea, is considered rare. Three such cases have been collected in the author's film library. The internal auditory canal may be normal, narrow, or absent. Labyrinthine abnormalities are common. Even the petrous pyramid is characteristically hypoplastic to the size of the facial nerve. When considering a cochlear implant, magnetic imaging can assist in identifying the presence of a cochlear nerve remnant. There may be a single labyrinthine cavity of varying size in the space normally taken by the inner ear structures.

Severe SNHL accompanies cochlear hypoplasia ("dwarf cochlea or microcochlea"). Such a hypoplastic cochlea has a normal shape and number of turns.

Cochlear dilation cases show irregular dilation of the cochlear lumen while the overall cochlear size and number of turns are usually normal.

Embrology Revisited

A simple axiom must be recalled. The inner ear is typically fully developed even to adult size by the end of the first trimester. In regard to the more subtle findings after the first trimester through the mid second trimester, it is a well-known fact that the otic capsule continues to grow until achieving full size, between the 5th and 6th months of gestation. Typically, normal ear morphology may result with more reduced dimensions, and these morphological changes can be shown on high resolution computerized tomograms (HRCT).[42]

Mondini Dysplasia (Figs 3–4 and 3–5)

The most common example of a bony malformation of the inner ear is Mondini dysplasia (as seen in imaging studies), in which there is incomplete development of the bony and membranous cochlea. This dysplasia was first described in 1791 by Carlo Mondini.[43] In Mondini's description, the semicircular canals were normal but the vestibule was somewhat larger than usual. Only the basal 1.5 coils of the cochlea were normal, and above them was found a wide cavity. It is now known that variations and degrees of severity are found in Mondini dysplasia.

SNHL resulting from Mondini dysplasia is due to dysgenesis of the end-organs and their neural elements. According to Paparella,[44] this condition is characterized by fewer than the normal 2.5 cochlear turns and an enlarged endolymphatic duct, and a deficient utriculoendolymphatic

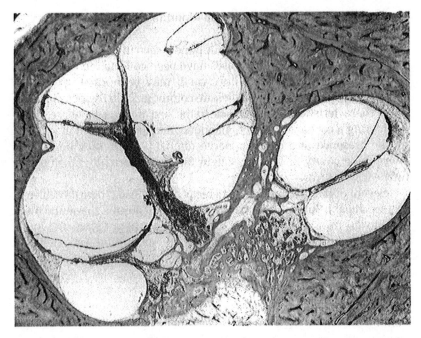

Fig 3-4.—Ultrastructural findings in a patient with residual high frequency hearing in Mondini dysplasia. (Courtesy of FH Linthicum, IR, MD, House Ear Institute, Los Angeles. Reprinted with permission.)

valve associated with the absence of endolymphatic hydrops. The state of a patient's hearing cannot be predicted upon the presence of Mondini malformation bone changes. It is thought that residual hearing varies with the degree of malformation; in some cases the individual may even have normal hearing. Furthermore, the hearing level may be maintained for weeks, months, or years before showing an increase in loss (Fig 3–6). Patient's with Mondini dysplasia characteristically demonstrate other temporal bone abnormalities that may cause progressive hearing loss. In those cases in which there is absence of the osseous spiral lamina between the apical and middle turns of the cochlea, a weakening of the basilar membrane results. This makes the membrane subject to rupture when there are increased pressures in the parallel from the cochlea aqueduct.[45]

Two elements are typically seen in radiographs of the Mondini malformation: (1) a normal or near normal basilar cochlea turn and (2) a single cochlear cavity in which the middle and apical cochlear coils are absent (Fig 3–5, A–C). In the latter situation, the spiral bone partition between the two

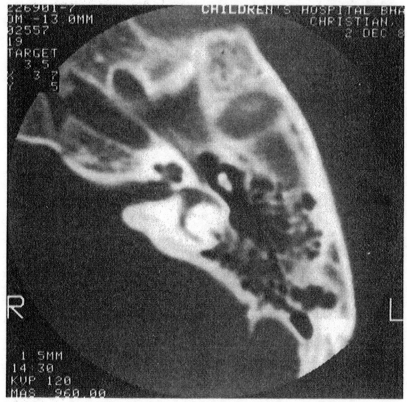

A

Fig 3-5.—A, Normal cochlear structures visualized by axial plane at 0°. B, CT scan evidence of Mondini dysplasia. The spirals of the cochlea are not identified, and the vestibule of the labyrinth is involved. C, Audiogram from patient whose CT scan of inner ear structures is shown in B. *(continued)*

top cochlear coils is absent and the modiolus is rudimentary. In such cases, the overall size of the cochlea may be small or normal.

It is generally acceptable that first trimester inner ear malformations may be diagnosed by HRCT. The physician would have to be aware of severe abnormalities that would occur in the first trimester and more subtle changes that can occur after this trimester. The development of the footplate with transformation from membrane to cartilage and/or bone would occur early in the first trimester. True fistulas that we have discovered were those in which the vestibular window contained only mem-

Fig 3-5. *(continued)*

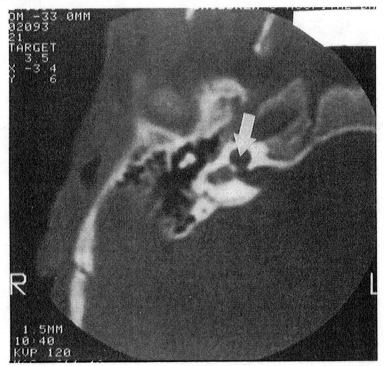

B

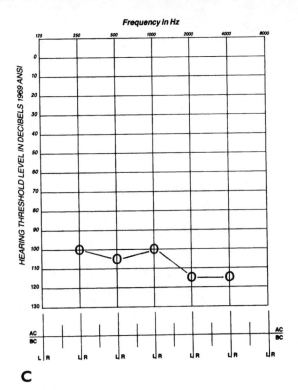

C

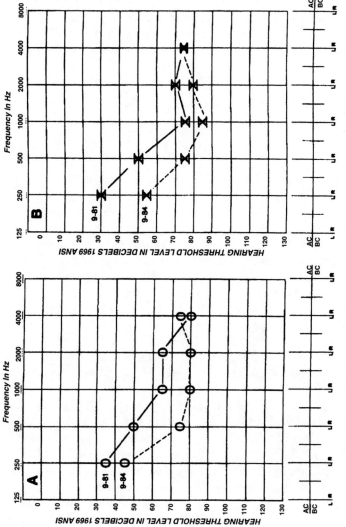

Fig 3-6.—A, Last audiogram (September 1984) of a 5-year-old child with a progressive hearing loss. Historically, the patient developed speech in two-word sentences at age 15 months, after which speech deteriorated. B, A younger sibling (age 3 years) of the patient in A has SNHL with a similar audiometric configuration. There is no family history or other findings to determine the cause of the hearing loss other than the fact it occurred in two siblings. Diagnosis: Recessive early onset deafness (recessive inheritance, delayed type).

85

brane and no cartilage in the footplate. Typically, a head injury early in life would tend to break this membrane and cause the fistula, and subsequently, the hearing loss.[46]

Patients with Mondini dysplasia and profound hearing impairment should be examined for ultra-audiometric hearing and the possibility that using special hearing aids that would transpose speech range frequencies into their residual hearing range. Since the basal turn of the cochlea remains intact in Mondini dysplasias, high frequency hearing should also be intact.

Vestibular Aqueduct Abnormalities

Many times, vestibular aqueduct abnormalities occur in conjunction with other radiographically visualized abnormalities. Congenital widening of the aqueduct may occur as a lone finding and be associated with hearing loss. This latter condition has been identified as the "large vestibular aqueduct syndrome."

It is important to differentiate the two morphologic patterns of cochlear malformations because the natural history of the hearing loss progression may differ. There can be a variance in the configuration and size of the vestibular aqueduct, especially of the posterior portion when one recognizes its embryological development. The anterior part forms first, and it takes a straight course paralleling the common crus of the semicircular canals to form the endolymphatic sac in the posterior cranial fossa. In normal circumstances, the changing configuration of the vestibular aqueduct due to completion of the capsule development is approximately 20 weeks. However, the posterior fossa continues to grow, and the most posterior portion of the vestibular aqueduct may change configuration, making the structure variable in location.

Okumura et al[47] suggested that the large vestibular aqueduct was the most common radiographically detectible malformation in patients with early onset SNHL. Occurring as an entity that includes inner defects, I doubt if this is true, since typically, there are abnormalities of other anatomical structures that occur with the abnormal vestibular aqueduct. Okumura found that the large vestibular aqueduct tends to affect high frequency hearing more than low frequency and that the incidents of sudden hearing loss were high. These sudden losses tended to be triggered by episodes such as minor head injury.

With such an incidence of sudden hearing loss, can the vestibular aqueduct syndrome predispose to perilabyrinthine fistula? Many have shown that with a large vestibular aqueduct the incidents of sudden hearing loss are relatively rare.[48-54]

A possible cause of this injury is the reflux of hyperosmolar fluid from the endolymphatic sac to the inner ear with resulting rupture of the perilabyrinthine membranes or membranous labyrinth, due to direct transmission of intracranial pressure to the inner ear through this enlarged vestibular aqueduct. Conceptually, this should primarily involve the labyrinthine membranes more than the perilabyrinthine windows. Furthermore, studies have not really proven this. More cases need to be evaluated in regard to this situation.

Cochlear Aqueduct Abnormalities

The cochlear aqueduct extends from the scala tympani of the basal turn of the cochlea adjacent to the round window to the inferior surface of the petrous bone adjacent to the anterior division of the jugular foramen. The width of the cochlear aqueduct at its infundibulum, where it is easily identified, has been found to be extremely variable. However, the base of the infundibulum tapers quickly in its intraosseous portion. Laterally, from this point, nonvisualization is common, although a minute lucency as it enters the basal turn of the cochlea is still considered normal.

Historically, the cochlear aqueduct was usually not seen on polytome studies.

HRCTs usually show identification of this structure. There is a variance of the enlargement of the internal funnel of the cochlear aqueduct that opens into the posterior fossa. One must evaluate the diameter of the structure from within the duct, typically at the level of the basal turn of the cochlea, the round window niche, and at the level of the posterior semicircular canal on the axial section. Valvassori et al[55] state that in 20% of ears with congenital anomalies of the otic capsule, the cochlear aqueduct is abnormally dilated. He also states that a dilated cochlear aqueduct occurs occasionally as an isolated defect. Typically, one has not been so concerned about the size of the aqueduct in relation to deafness, as in relation to the cause of a labyrinthine emergence of cerebrospinal fluid (CSF), which can sometimes occur during stapedectomy from otosclerosis or congenital footplate fixation. In recent decades the stapes gusher has been thought to be due to abnormal connections between the internal auditory canal and vestibule, rather than that of the enlarged or patent cochlear aqueduct, though the latter may be known to cause an oozing rather than a gushing.[56,57] The cochlear aqueduct is abnormally dilated in about 20% of ear and congenital anomalies of the otic capsule.

Internal Auditory Canal Abnormalities

When labyrinthine hypoplasia is present, as in Michel dysplasia, it is usual for the internal auditory canals to be narrowed to the size of the facial nerve, if the latter is present.

Nonenlargement of the internal auditory canal is seen in neurofibromatosis, RP, and osteogenesis imperfecta.

The axis of the internal auditory canal in the fetus is directed backward and downward. The internal auditory canals in adults normally point medially.

The importance of detecting the enlargement of the internal auditory canal is its association with spontaneous CSF leak and gusher, especially during stapes surgery.

Typically, one should get an HRCT scan prior to surgery for congenital fixation, since hearing results with stapedectomy following perilymphatic fluid gushers are frequently poor. Dilatation of the internal auditory canal, especially when there is little or no space between the lateral end of the canal and the vestibular window and the inner ear appears abnormal, would tend to contraindicate a stapedectomy.

The size of the internal auditory canal is extremely variable. It is considered stenotic if it is 3 mm or less in width or height.[42]

Vestibule and Semicircular Canals

The lateral semicircular canal is the structure involved most commonly in labyrinthine malformations. It may be absent or may be a mere vestibular projection.[58]

In our study of the cause of SNHL where the structures of the inner ear appeared grossly normal, in cases with SNHL we looked for unique and minute differences in the structures of the inner ear. A shortened lateral semicircular canal (on axial view) was the most common finding in this study.[42]

Phyllogenetically, the superior and posterior semicircular canals are first found in *Myxinoidea* (hagfish). In later development, for example, in the *Alasmobranchii* (spine shark) the lateral semicircular canal is present. According to Jackler and Luxford,[59] approximately 40% of ears with malformed cochleas will have accompanying dysplasia of the lateral semicircular canal. Ears with malformations that are limited to the vestibular system may have normal or near normal hearing.

Radiology and Inner Ear Defects
of Congenital Inheritance

The association of hearing impairment and malformation of the ear has been obvious for some time, and the fact that such malformations may be among the causes of congenital hearing loss has been known for over a century.[60] Polytomography and CT scanning have made it possible to clinically identify a wide spectrum of ear anomalies; however, malformations of the inner ear were never considered rare. As mentioned, the most common abnormality is that of the semicircular canals. It is followed in frequency by a combined deformity of the cochlea, vestibule, and semicircular canals. Malformed semicircular canals are either narrow and show an atypical course, or are shortened and wide.[61] In Mondini dysplasia, variance of the anatomical defect is the rule, as incomplete and minor defects of the disorder may be associated with little or no auditory or vestibular dysfunction, and severe forms may occur with complete dysfunction. Seemingly, most any inner ear defect could be regarded as a variation of Mondini dysplasia.

Incidence

Although it cannot be definitely concluded from radiographic studies that inner ear defects are the cause of a hearing loss, in a histopathological study by Suehiro and Sando,[62] most anomalies of the inner ear appear to be associated with hearing problems (41 cases in 43, or 95%).

Heretofore, there have been no established reports of inner ear defects occurring with viral lesions causing a congenital SNHL, for example, rubella or CMV. More recently, Bauman et al[41] reported a case of bilateral temporal bone anomalies in a child with symptomatic congenital CMV having SNHL. They performed further studies on other children with CMV and hearing loss, and out of the next five children with the condition, one patient had severe bilateral temporal bone dysplasias with a small cochlea. Other findings were present. In other cases, measurements were established and subtle findings such as shortened cochlea dimensions, narrow vestibules, and narrow lateral canals were identified. Such results, they concluded, could indicate that congenital CMV infection causes anomalies or growth disturbances of the temporal bone.

A high incidence of Mondini dysplasia has been found in Pendred's syndrome,[63] Klippel-Feil syndrome, trisomy syndromes, and DiGeorge syndrome.[32]

Sporadic Inner Ear Defects

Sporadic inner ear deformities may be those in which the hearing loss is produced either by a mutational gene (usually dominant) or by an X-linked dominant gene. Medical monitoring over several generations may be necessary before the mendelian mechanism involved can be established exactly. The possibility of prenatal intoxicant or drug use cannot be absolutely excluded, as family reticence could be functioning. The incidence of sporadic inner ear defects clearly illustrates the clinical value of radiography in determining a suspected genetic cause for a SNHL. In cases in which only inner ear defects are found, there is a strong inclination to assume that the origin is genetic, as it is in such conditions occurring in association with syndromes.

Hereditary Progressive SNHL

Therapeutic considerations have been to little or no avail in hereditary progressive SNHL, and steps need to be taken to cope with the consequences. Previous audiograms, if available, must be obtained so that the physician can determine if the hearing loss is progressive. The original baseline audiogram is invaluable, not only to confirm the progression, but also to establish accurate thresholds. It is well-documented that establishment of a diagnosis, audiometric testing, and evaluation of recent hearing and learning performance in children who are hearing-impaired (by the mother or educator) are all of utmost importance in determining whether there has been a progression in hearing loss.

It is possible for a progressive SNHL to become stable or for a fluctuating loss to become progressive. Considering all children with a SNHL, there is a high incidence of progressive losses (author's statistics). For this reason, it is imperative that children with SNHL be monitored. When progressive loss is suspected, the patient requires weekly monitoring. If progression is suspected but has not yet been manifested, such as in cases of meningitis or CMV disease, the hearing should be tested every 3 months. All children with SNHL should be tested for hearing every 6 months. This monitoring procedure is carried out up to the age of 8 years. After that age, each patient should be evaluated according to his or her individual needs, but at least once a year. If the hearing has remained stable, a yearly audiogram may be adequate.

Since the specific course of management should be directed by a professional who knows the pathophysiology of SNHL and is in a position to institute the appropriate treatment, it must be prescribed by a physician.

Early progressive hearing losses can be documented clinically. In view of the difficulties in detection of SNHL in early infancy, however, audiometric and clinical determination of the progressive features of hearing impairment is rarely possible. Nevertheless, there is clinical evidence from some parents that their children were developing words when, at or after the age of 1 year, a deterioration of speech and language occurred. Such historical documentation is indicative of progressive SNHL occurring during this period and is considered a "high risk factor" for hereditary delayed SNHL. It is important that true words be reported, rather than "babbling" words such as "Mama," "Dada," and "bye-bye" that occur in all babies around the age of 6 months.

From data available from animal studies, it is suspected that sound deprivation as a result of the loss of the organ of Corti has an irreversible effect on the development of the auditory pathways.[64-67] Furthermore, the earlier the anatomical loss of the inner ear occurs in the development of an animal, the greater the anatomical effect on the central auditory pathways. This presumption has immense clinical application: It is imperative to diagnose the presence of a hearing loss in neonates and initiate amplification early.

POSTDIAGNOSIS IMPLEMENTATIONS

It must be pointed out that biological inheritance alone does not make the total person; environmental factors can influence inherited traits. Every person inherits a basic mental ability that determines his or her capacity to learn. However, a child's environment may also determine the opportunities to develop this capacity. Children with hereditary SNHL can learn speech and language with early identification and stimulation. Therefore, the amount a child may learn depends on both inherited ability and environment—that is, parents, community, schools, and so forth. Ling and Nienhuys[68] have enumerated other psychoeducational variables that affect a child's ability to learn. It is important to differentiate, from the information gleaned by a thorough history, inherited delayed SNHL from inherited congenital SNHL. We have found that children with a severe to profound inherited delayed SNHL may develop good language skills even when a severe loss was identified as late as age 17 months. This was most likely due to the fact that sound was audible in the early months of life and, consequently, some development of auditory perception occurred. Such children should be given the opportunity to develop speech and language skills with normally hearing children; that is, they should be exposed to the auditory-verbal method of teaching children with hearing impairment. On the other hand, when confirmation of an inherited severe to profound hearing loss occurring before birth can be made, we have found that progress in the development of speech and language skills is slower and more difficult to achieve. Children born with severe to profound hearing loss can do as well as children who lose their hearing after birth, provided the loss is identified early, preferably in the first year of life or, ideally, at birth.

It can be stipulated that, for development to proceed efficaciously, early evaluation of learning abilities and determination of the presence of communicative disorders (hearing, speech, language) is needed. Children with severe-to-profound hearing loss who develop good speech and language must continue to be monitored, even into the teenage years, to avoid regression of speech.

Proof of subsequent impairments in language development resulting from mild to moderate hearing loss has not yet been established. Children with such losses should be monitored twice a year in the early school years for both progression of hearing loss and retardation of speech and language skills.

REFERENCES

1. Gorlin RJ, Toriello HV, Cohen M Jr. *Hereditary Hearing Loss and Its Syndromes.* New York, NY: Oxford University Press; 1995:10-11.
2. Finley WH. Genetic screening: an overview. *Alabama Med Sci.* 1982;19: 147-150.
3. Bergstrom L, Hemenway WG, Downs MP. A high-risk registry to find congenital deafness. *Otolaryngol Clin North Am.* 1971; 4:369-399.
4. Konigsmark BW, Gorlin RJ. *Genetic and Metabolic Deafness.* Philadelphia, Pa: WB Saunders; 1976:1.
5. Schein JD, Delt MT. *The deaf population of the United States.* Silver Spring, Md: National Association of the Deaf; 1974.
6. Rizer, FM. *Current diagnosis and management of SNHL in children.* (Handout). *American Academy of Otolaryngology—Head and Neck Surgery;* 1995.
7. Pappas DG. A study of the high risk registry for sensorineural hearing impairment. *Otolaryngol Head Neck Surg.* 1983;91:41-44.
8. Paparella MM. Differential diagnosis of childhood deafness. In: Bess FH, ed. *Childhood Deafness—Causation, Assessment and Management.* New York, NY: Grune & Stratton; 1977:3-18.
9. Finley SC. Genetic counseling. *Alabama J Med Sci.* 1982;19:165-168.
10. Stern C. *Principles of Human Genetics.* 2nd ed. San Francisco, Ca: WH Freeman; 1960:454.

11. Nance WE, Sweeney A. Genetic factors in deafness of early life. *Otolaryngol Clin North Am*. 1975;8:19-48.
12. Fraser GR. The genetics of congenital deafness. *Otolaryngol Clin North Am*. 1971;4:227-247.
13. McKusick VA. Diseases of the genome. *JAMA*. 1984; 252:1041-1048.
14. Nance WE. Questions about genetics. *Our Kids Magazine*. Alexander Graham Bell Association for the Deaf, Fall 1983.
15. Nance WE, Setleff RC, McLeod A, et al. X-linked mixed deafness with congenital fixation of the stapedial footplate and perilymphatic gushers. *Birth Defects*. 1971;7:64-69.
16. Nyhan WL. Cytogenetic diseases. *Clin Symp*. 1983;35:2-32.
17. Clements PR, Bates MVA, Hafer M. Variability within Down's syndrome (trisomy 21): empirically observed sex differences in IQs. *Ment Retard*. 1976;14:30-31.
18. Saxon SA, Witriol E. Down's syndrome and intellectual development. *J Pediatr Psychol*. 1976;1:4-47.
19. Mahoney G, Glover A, Finger I. Relationship between language and sensorimotor development of Down syndrome and nonretarded children. *Am J Ment Defic*. 1981;86:21-27.
20. Greenwald CA, Leonard LB. Communicative and sensorimotor development of Down's syndrome children. *Am J Ment Def*. 1979;84:296-303.
21. Rynders JE, Behlin KL, Horrobin JM. Performance characteristics of preschool Down's syndrome children receiving augmented or repetitive instructions. *Am J Ment Defic*. 1979;84:67-73.
22. Balkany TJ, Mischke RE, Downs MP, Jafek BW. Ossicular abnormalities in Down's syndrome. *Otolaryngol Head Neck Surg*. 1979;87:372-384.
23. Brooks DN, Wooley H, Kanjilal GC. Hearing loss and middle ear disorders in patients with Down's syndrome (mongolism). *Am J Ment Defic Res*. 1972;16: 21-29.
24. Balkany TJ, Mischke RE, Downs MP, Jafek BW, Krajicek MJ. Hearing loss in Down's syndrome. *Clin Pediatr*. 1977;18:175-181.
25. Igarashi M, Takahaski M, Alford BR, Johnson PE. Inner ear morphology in Down's syndrome. *Acta Otolaryngol*. 1977;83:175-181.
26. Keiser H, Montague J, Wold D, et al. Hearing loss of Down syndrome adults. *Am J Ment Defic*. 1981;85:467-472.
27. Pappas DG, Flexor CG, Shackelford L. Otological and habilitative management of children with Down's syndrome. *Laryngoscope*. September 1994;104: 1065-1075.
28. Kos AO, Schuknecht HF, Singer JD. Temporal bone studies in 13-15 and 18 trisomy syndromes. *Arch Otolaryngol*. 1966;83:57-63.
29. Sando I, Bergstrom L, Wood RP, Hemenway WG. Temporal bone findings in trisomy 18 syndrome. *Arch Otolaryngol*. 1970;91:552-559.
30. Maniglia AJ, Wolff D, Herques AJ. Congenital deafness in 13-15 and 18 trisomy syndrome. *Arch Otolaryngol*. 1970;92:181-188.
31. Black FO, Sando I, Wagner, JA, Hemenway WG. Middle and inner ear abnormalities. *Arch Otolaryngol*. 1970;92:181-188.

32. Schuknecht HF. Mondini dysplasia: a clinical and pathological study. *Ann Otol Rhinol Laryngol.* 1980;89(suppl 65):3-23.
33. Paparella MM. Mondini's deafness: a review of histopathology. *Ann Otol Rhinol Laryngol.* 1980;89(suppl 67):1-10.
34. Lindsay JR, Caruthers DG, Hemenway WG, Harrison S. Inner ear pathology following maternal rubella. *Ann Otol Rhinol Laryngol.* 1953;62:1201-1217.
35. Hart C, Naunton R. The ototoxicity of chloroquine phosphate. *Arch Otolaryngol.* 1964;80:407-412.
36. Schuknecht HF. *Pathology of the Ear.* Cambridge, Ma: Harvard University Press; 1976:197.
37. Rubin R. Development of the inner ear of the mouse: a radioautographic study of terminal mitosis. *Acta Otolaryngol.* 1967(suppl 220):1-44.
38. Bosher SK, Hallpike ES. Observations on the histogenesis of the inner ear degeneration of the deaf white cat and its possible relationship to the etiology of certain unexplained varieties of human congenital deafness. *J Laryngol Otol.* 1966;60:222-235.
39. Mikelian D, Ruhin RJ. Development of hearing in the normal CBA-J mouse. *Acta Otolaryngol.* 1964;59:451-461.
40. Anderson H, Henricson B, Lundquist P-G, et al. Genetic hearing impairment in the Dalmatian dog. *Acta Otolaryngol.* 1968;(suppl 232):26-33.
41. Bauman NH, Kirby-Keyser LJ, Dolan KD, et al. Mondini dysplasia and congenital cytomegalovirus infection. *J Peds.* January 1994:71-78.
42. Pappas DG, Simpson LC, McKenzie, RA, Royal S. High-resolution computed tomography: determination of the cause of pediatric sensorineural hearing loss. *Laryngoscope.* June 1990;100(6):564-569.
43. Mondini C. Anatomica surdi nati sectio. *The DeBononiems: Institute of Science and Art and Commentary of the Banoniae Academy.* 1791;7:419-431.
44. Paparella, MM. Mondini's deafness: a review of histopathology. *Ann Otol Rhinol Laryngol.* 1980;89(suppl 67):1-10.
45. Ibid.
46. Pappas, DG, Simpson, LC, Godwin, GH. Perilymphatic fistula in children with preexisting sensorineural hearing loss. *Laryngoscope.* May 1988;98(5):507-510.
47. Okumura T, Takahashi H, Honjo I, Takagi A, Mitamura K. Sensorineural hearing loss in patients with large vestibular aqueduct. *Laryngoscope.* March 1995;105(3):289-294.
48. Mafee MF, Selis JE, Yannias DA, et al. Congenital sensorineural hearing loss. *Radiology.* 1984;150:427-434.
49. Hill JH, Freint AJ, Mafee MF. Enlargement of the vestibular aqueduct. *Ann Otolaryngol.* 1984;5:411-414.
50. Emmett JR. The large vestibular aqueduct syndrome. *Am J Otol.* 1985;6:387-415.
51. Levenson MJ, Parisier SC, Jacobs M, et al. The large vestibular aqueduct syndrome in children. *Arch Otolaryngol Head Neck Surg.* 1989;115:54-58.
52. Jackler RK, De La Cruz A. The large vestibular aqueduct syndrome, *Laryngoscope.* 1989;99:1238-1243.

53. Urman SM, Tabot JM. Otic capsule dysplasia: clinical and CT Findings. *Radiography*. 1990;10:823-838.
54. Arcand P, Desrosiers M, Dube J, et al. The large vestibular aqueduct syndrome and sensorineural hearing loss in pediatric population. *J Otolaryngol*. 1991;20: 247-250.
55. Valvassori GE, Mafee MF, Carter BL. *Imaging of the Head and Neck*. New York, NY: Thieme Medical Publishers, Inc.; 1995:51.
56. Glasscock ME. The stapes gusher. *Arch Otolaryngol*. 1973;98:82-91.
57. Schuchnecht HF, Reisser C. The morphologic basis for perilymph gushers and oozers. *Adv Oto Rhino Laryngol*. 1988;39:1-12.
58. Gensen J. Congenital anomalies of the inner ear. *Rad Clin North Am*. 1974;12: 473-482.
59. Jackler RK, Luxford WM, eds. Congenital malformations of the inner ear, *Laryngoscope*. 1987;97(supp 40, No. 3, Pt 2):2-14.
60. Jensen J. Malformations of the inner ear in deaf children. *Acta Radiologica*. 1969;8(suppl 286):11-84.
61. Reisner K. Tomography in inner and middle ear malformation. *Radiology*. 1969;92:11-20.
62. Suehiro S, Sando I: Congenital anomalies of the inner ear. *Ann Otol Rhinol Laryngol*. 1979;88(suppl 59):1-24.
63. Illum P. The Mondini type of cochlear malformation: a survey of the literature. *Arch Otolaryngol*. 1972;96:305-311.
64. Webster DB, Webster M. Mouse brainstem auditory nuclei development. *Ann Otol Rhinol Laryngol*. 1960;89(suppl 68):254-256.
65. Levi-Montalcini R. Development of the acoustico-vestibular centers in chick embryo in the absence of the afferent root fibers and descending fiber tracts. *J Comp Neurol*. 1949;91:209-234.
66. Jackson JK, Rubel EW. Rapid transneural degeneration following cochlear removal in the chick. *Anat Rec*. 1976;184:434.
67. Parks TN, Robinson J. The effects of otocyst removal on the development of chick brain stem auditory nuclei. *Anat Rec*. 1976;184:497.
68. Ling D, Nienhnys TG. The deaf child: habilitation with and without a cochlear implant. *Ann Otol Rhinol Laryngol*. 1983;92:593-598.

CHAPTER

4

Hearing Loss Associated With Perinatal Infections

An investigator needs facts, and not legends or rumours.

It is the first quality of a criminal investigator the he should see through a disguise.

The Hound of the Baskervilles
Sherlock Holmes

Of all known causes of hearing loss in neonates and children, perhaps the most difficult to confirm are those resulting from infectious agents. Until the invention of the electron microscope in the late 1930s, viruses could not be identified and were studied by the pathogenic effects they caused in infected tissues or by the damage created when injected into animals. The innovation of electron microscopy made it possible to examine, in detail, the structure of viruses, their relationship to cells, and the reactions of cells invaded by them. In recent decades, methods for growing cells in culture and making monolayer cultures have been introduced. These developments have aided the exact quantitative studies of viral multiplication and the action of specific antibodies on virus growth. As a result of these discoveries, specific laboratory tests (such as agglutination tests) provide information that is helpful not only in making a diagnosis, but also in relating a previous infection with its infectious agent, for example, the agglutination titer for rubella. When the practical results of the advances in virology (such as the polio and rubella vaccines) and their beneficial effects on the health of mankind are considered, their contribution is second in importance only to the discovery of antibiotics.[1]

A virus is a unique infectious agent in that it has a relatively simple chemical composition, is smaller than other infectious agents, lacks enzymes for energy metabolism, multiplies intracellularly, and appears to have no life of its own outside of cells. The cells that become infected by a virus develop properties different from those of normal cells. They may respond to the infection in one of the following ways: degeneration and death, transformation into a new growth (neoplasia), or survival without transformation but with evidence of the presence of the virus.

The role of viruses as the causative agents in hearing loss has not been clearly defined. It is definitely known, however, that the congenitally acquired virus of rubella and cytomegalovirus (CMV) are linked to hearing impairment, the latter virus having been identified in the sensory organ of the inner ear. Definitive evidence of the destruction of the organ of Corti as a result of rubella infection is one of association of clinical findings, as the virus has never been detected in the inner ear.

There is little evidence to support the indictment of the rubella and CMV virus as the cause of acquired hearing loss. Certainly, acquired hearing loss occurring in the postnatal years as a result of rubella or CMV infection is almost nonexistent. The mumps virus has been implicated as a cause of unilateral hearing loss; however, previous temporal bone studies in such cases have shown only what appears to have been evidence of a viral reaction.[2] In cases of acquired hearing loss, a viral cause may be suspected on the basis of a recent history of an upper respiratory infection or flu-type symptoms, the absence of bacteria, or serological evidence of recent infection (seroconversion or significant rises in specific antibody titers) to a particular virus. Although congenital hearing loss induced by viral infection has been proved, a viral cause is difficult to ascertain in cases of acquired hearing impairment.

CLASSIFICATIONS OF INFECTIONS

Characteristics of chronic prenatal infections include, in addition to their chronic (and often recurrent) nature in the mother, the ability of the agent to cross the placenta or its membranes, and the ability to produce persistent infections in the fetus. Included in this group are the so-called TORCHS agents: toxoplasma, rubella, cytomegalovirus (CMV), herpes simplex virus, hepatitis B virus, and syphilis. The high risk for hearing impairment from rubella, CMV, and syphilis are well-recognized, and their impact on the outcome of the pregnancy and on the long-term morbidity of the offspring is well-known.

Another group of perinatal infections is characterized by an acute, self-limiting course that may be suppressed by the body's defensive mechanisms, and which is followed by a complete or partial immunity to reinfection. According to Stagno and coworkers,[3] early in gestation, when the infection overwhelms the patient or is severe, it may result in termination of the pregnancy. When incurred late in gestation, the degree of infection in the newborn may range from subclinical manifestations to severe multi-organ disease. The explanations for how some of these infectious agents cause hearing impairment have been speculative. The relationship between sensorimotor functioning and language development in acute cases has not been explored to the extent that it has been in cases of chronic perinatal infections. Some of the more common infectious agents in the prenatal group include viruses such as echo, coxsackie A and B, measles, varicella, mumps, and influenza viruses, and bacteria such as group B streptococcus and *Escherichia coli*.

SCREENING FOR CAUSES OF HEARING LOSS

The proportion of cases of SNHL found to be associated with viral infections in pediatric patients has increased since the advent of viral screening procedures.[3] It has been estimated that neonatal hearing loss caused by a virus occurs once in some 2700 births (author's statistics). Therefore, to routinely screen for viral agents during the neonatal period may not be cost efficient. However, when a neonate fails a screening test for hearing, viral studies should be initiated. The correct diagnosis of a postviral infection hearing loss could avoid the consequences of an incorrect diagnosis, such as a hereditary SNHL.

Historically, determination of immunoglobulin M (IgM) levels in serum collected at birth from the umbilical cord has been described previously as a screening method for the detection of infection.[4] Another screening test performed in the past for detection of chronic perinatal infections, the rheumatoid factor (RF) agglutination test, yields a high percentage (greater than 50%) of false-negative results[5]; the number of false-positive results is very small. The levels of these antibodies (IgM and RF) are not used routinely to screen for infectious agents because of the high incidence of false-negative results.

A urine specimen taken from a neonate suspected of having a hearing loss and inoculated into tissue culture tubes is the most sensitive test for CMV. Positive findings from such a test performed during the first 3 weeks of life is strong presumptive evidence that hearing loss is the result of this virus. If CMV is first isolated after the neonatal period, however, its diagnostic value is severely limited, since 10 to 40% of normal infants in the United States acquire CMV infection between 2 and 6 months of age, according to S Stagno et al.[6] Excretion of CMV in the urine continues for months, and even years, and decreases with time.[6] Despite continued viral excretion, most infected patients appear to be in good health and may develop normally.

During the time that congenital rubella was prevalent it was noticed that 50 to 65%[3,7] of cases were asymptomatic, and that certain laboratory examinations had to be initiated when the mother had a positive history of exposure or when routine screening yielded suspicious findings and the child failed a hearing screening test (Table 4–1). A throat viral culture from the infant and serial determination of specific antibody titers from both infant and mother are also indicated.

For maternal syphilis, the routine Venereal Disease Research Laboratory (VDRL) test is used and, if positive, is followed by a fluorescent treponema antibody test (FTA-ABS) on the mother's serum. Subclinical signs are not apparent in approximately 50% of all neonates infected with syphilis.[8]

Toxoplasmosis is not known to cause SNHL.[9,10] Seventy five percent of the neonates infected by toxoplasma exhibit an absence of symptoms.[3]

Cytomegalovirus (CMV)

Although occurring in only 0.5 to 2.4%[11-13] of all live births, CMV infection is the most frequent viral intrauterine infection. This herpeslike virus characteristically forms an intracellular nuclear inclusion.[14]

Some neonates have birth defects that can be detected only by specific testing. Hearing loss is prevalent among infants infected by CMV; indeed, CMV infection is the leading cause of virus-related SNHL in infants. However, 90% of the infants infected with CMV are asymptomatic at birth and appear normal[3]; only 10% have clinically apparent disease at

Table 4–1. Diagnostic Aids

Cytomegalovirus (CMV) infection	Isolation of virus from urine within first 2 weeks of life
Rubella	Isolation of virus from throat (and stool, conjunctiva, or urine) within 1 month of age
	Serial determination of antibody (hemagglutination inhibition) between 3 and 9 months of age
Syphilis	Darkfield examination of lesions if present
	Antibody determination with both reagin (VDRL) and fluorescent antibody (FTA-ABS) tests
Toxoplasmosis	Isolation of Toxoplasma gondii from placenta,
	CSF, or blood; serial determination of IgG antibody (immunofluorescence) between 1 and 6 months of age; determination of IgM antibody in cord serum
Hepatitis B	Serial determination of hepatitis B surface antigen (HBsAg), antibody to the hepatitis B surface antigen (anti-HBs), and antibody to the hepatitis B core antigen (anti-HBc)
Herpes simplex	Isolation of virus from skin vesicles and conjunctiva (presence of virus throat, CSF, and stool also possible)

Adapted from Stagno S, et al.[13] Used with permission of March of Dimes-Birth Defects Foundation.

birth. Children affected with this form of infection are usually at high risk of having disabilities that will significantly impair their development.[12,15] Pass and colleagues,[16] in a study of 34 patients with systemic CMV infection at birth, reported that 10 of these patients died as neonates. Of the remaining 24 surviving patients, all but two had evidence of CNS or auditory handicaps. Microcephaly was present in 16 patients (70%), mental retardation in 14 (61%), and hearing impairment in 7 (30%).

In stark contrast, infants with the asymptomatic (subclinical) form of congenital CMV infection appeared normal at birth, but on screening were found to excrete CMV in their urine. Pathological studies have suggested that hearing impairment occurs in between 7 and 17% of the cases[6] and that it may be caused by a focal viral infection of the cochlea (Table 4–1).[17-19]

SNHL Associated With CMV

Infants with hearing loss produced by subclinical CMV infection have demonstrated inconsistency in the patterns and frequency of auditory impairments. Some have been found to have mild to profound bilateral SNHL with impairment in both high and low frequencies; some have asymmetrical involvement; and some have unilateral hearing loss.[20-23]

CMV infections of the inner ear cause either partial or total cochlear and labyrinthine end-organ destruction.[21] Abnormal vestibular findings have been confirmed by tests in some patients with congenital CMV infection.[20] These patients exhibited a delay in gross motor skills (walking, standing), but their fine motor skills (grasping) were normal. The subnormal intelligence, behavioral problems, and learning disabilities in these patients are not conclusive evidence, and only a small number have shown signs of mental deficiency.[15,16] Nonetheless, the possibility remains that a recurrence of the infection might cause damage to the brain or perceptual organs that would be manifested with advancing age. Such damage is reflected in the high incidence of progressive hearing loss (in 19 of 35 patients) found in patients with subclinical CMV infection following a period of hearing level stability. Whether or not the virus remains dormant in the inner ear and later becomes active again is not known.

Once the hearing loss is confirmed, close audiological monitoring is necessary because of the progressive nature of the disease. In addition to pure tone sound field audiometry, aided sound field testing is recommended. This is particularly important in monitoring the educational management of these children. Inconsistent responses to sounds that should be audible (based on aided audiograms) may indicate presence of a risk factor for central auditory processing. Intellectual retardation is not uncommon in some patients with congenital CMV infection. CNS defects must be sought for during the educational process.

Infants and children with asymmetrical hearing caused by CMV infection should be tested every month for 6 months because progression of the hearing loss seems to be prevalent in this group. The consequences of this prognosis must be dealt with in terms of habilitation management. Aided and unaided audiometric testing is recommended every 6 months until the child is 4 years old, when the hearing levels appear to stabilize.

Fluctuating hearing loss has not been reported in cases of hearing impairment induced by CMV infection. SNHL caused by CMV infection is not treatable; early and continuous audiological management and early introduction to ongoing educational management are essential.

Systemic Immunity to CMV

Although it is generally accepted that most viral infections are a one-time manifestation, systemic immunity to CMV has continued to be questioned. Some of this suspicion may have been eliminated by the report of Harris and colleagues.[25] In their study, these investigators injected the inner ears of animals that had high serum levels of guinea pig CMV (GPCMV) antibodies with GPCMV serum and found no evidence of significant hearing loss in the animals 8 days later. This might lead to the conclusion that the animals were protected against CMV by immunity. Such a judgment should be approached with caution, however, since the involvement and responsibility of CMV in hearing loss are still relatively speculative. That is, not all humans infected by CMV will develop hearing loss. Although the total number of subjects is small, the documented statistics are significant: 17% of subjects in subclinical infections[21] and 30% in clinically manifested infections[16] developed hearing loss.

Pathophysiology of CMV Infection

In a case of subclinical CMV infection, routine light microscopy revealed edema and inflammatory reactions in the plasma and mononuclear cells of the vestibule and cochlea. Incidental cells, showing the typical CMV intracellular nuclear inclusion, were found in Reissner's membrane and in the stria vascularis of the cochlea, but were not otherwise identified among the critical structures of the temporal bone and inner ear.[21] When these same inner ear cell structures were studied by means of anticomplement immunofluorescence, viral antigens were found to be widely distributed within the cochlea. This damaged cell reaction was not only cytopathologically detectable by means of standard histological staining procedures, but was also clearly manifested among the cells of the organ of Corti and the neurons of the spiral ganglion (Fig 4–1).

Rubella

Acquired rubella is a mild disease of children and young adults caused by a virus and manifested by a rash, rarely lasting more than 3 days, that starts on the face and spreads to the trunk and extremities. This rash is characteristically preceded by tender lymphadenopathy. Congenital rubella, on the other hand, is not a benign disease. Fetal infections caused by the rubella virus may result in hearing impairment, cardiac lesions, LBW (less than 2600 grams), eye defects (particularly cataracts), growth retardation, thrombocytopenic purpura, hepatosplenomegaly, hepatitis, and CNS defects such as psychomotor retardation, macrocephaly, encephalitis, or aseptic meningitis.[26,27] Indeed, the sequelae of congenital rubella gave impetus to the development of a vaccine against this virus.

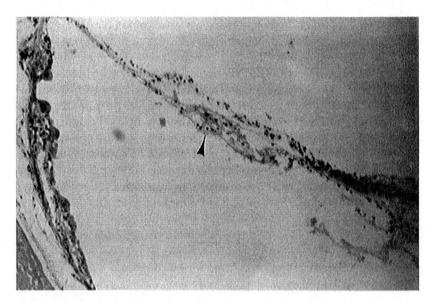

Fig 4-1.—Reissner's membrane. Photomicrograph (× 5000) showing inclusion body (arrow) in infant who died from systemic CMV infection. (Courtesy of Sergio B. Stagno, MD. Birmingham, Ala.)

Clinical Immunology

In those patients who contract the natural disease, neutralizing antibodies and the cells involved in cell-mediated immunity (CMI) are both detectable after infection. The neutralizing antibodies provide protection against the disease on reexposure. CMI may be important in recovery from the disease, but its role as a protective agent against reinfections is unclear.[28]

The RA 27/3 (rubella) vaccine usually induces a fourfold rise in titer in those who have been vaccinated with it. Reinfection with rubella following inoculation appears to be infrequent.[29]

Prenatal rubella does not produce high antibody titers in all children, and there appears to be a gradual loss of such antibodies, resulting in very low levels after 3 or 4 years of age; alternatively, the antibodies may disappear altogether (serofast negative).[30] There may be no increase in the agglutination titers in prenatally infected patients even after the rubella vaccine is administered. Consequently, it is possible to confirm a diagnosis of congenital rubella in children over 2 years of age by determining the presence of a low rubella antibody titer that does not respond to the rubella vaccine.

Incidence of Rubella

Epidemiologically, rubella has appeared in cycles of approximately 5 to 7 years. Goodhill[31] stated that reports emanating from the 1940 severe and widespread rubella epidemic in Australia brought worldwide attention to this disease as a cause of hearing impairment, a previously unrecognized sequela. Additional information made available by Goodhill revealed that Gregg's original report[26] was followed in 1946 by another report giving the statistics of 111 cases of hearing impairment resulting from rubella infection in 130 patients.

The prevalence and severity of congenital defects resulting from rubella infection varied in each epidemic. However, studies are consistent in reporting rubella to be most detrimental when the infection occurs in the first 3 months of pregnancy; similar, but less severe, defects are found when the infection occurs during the second trimester; and defects are rarely seen from infection in the third trimester (although rubella may act as a nonteratogenic but severe, chronic infection in the third trimester).[7]

Before the vaccine became available in the United States in 1968, 80 to 90% of the population had been infected by the time of adulthood. Different strategies have been chosen in various countries to prevent congenital rubella by vaccination. The strategy applied in the United States has been to immunize preschool and elementary school children, with the aim of preventing "pools" of rubella epidemics. This strategy has been successful.

Pathophysiology of Rubella

Studies of the temporal bone subsequent to rubella infection have demonstrated a degeneration of the organ of Corti, as manifested by a cochleosaccular change such as is seen in cases of Scheibe's syndrome. The degree of pathology caused by the arrest of development varies in each case and is reflected in the clinical variation in hearing loss.[32,33] Anomalies of the middle ear are found less frequently and an anomaly of the stapes due to cartilaginous fixation of the footplate was found in one case.[34] Although not described in the literature, another bony anomaly, Mondini dysplasia, has been mentioned in some cases of congenital rubella. One theory proposed as an explanation of bony defects in cases of congenital rubella is that damage occurs to the embryonic inner ear during the formation of the bony cochlea in the first trimester.

Temporal bone studies have never demonstrated the rubella virus in the cochlea, possibly because these studies have not included electron microscopic studies for intracellular changes.

SNHL Associated With Rubella

Many reports describe a "flat" configuration to the audiogram revealing hearing loss secondary to rubella; however, variation in hearing patterns seems to be more common. Falling contours in the high frequencies followed by declining contours in the low frequencies have been reported. Barr and Lundstrom [35] and Borton and Stark [36] also state that trough-shaped configurations are commonly seen. In most of their cases, they found variations in the severity of the hearing loss along with a lack of symmetry of hearing. In addition, they also observed total hearing loss.

Progression of the hearing loss associated with rubella is common. It is not clear if the progression is time-related, occurring only in the first 3 years of life, or if it represents an ongoing process. However, seropositive neonates with defects have been reported to develop other defects by 6 to 8 years of age.[37] This would support the existence of progression and stress the importance of long-term audiological follow-up.

Excluding severe mental handicaps, 33% of the children with congenital rubella were found to be poor learners and 66% had satisfactory scholastic records.[38] In comparing children with rubella induced hearing loss with those having hearing losses from other causes, no differences were observed across a wide range of educational, psychological, and communication variables.[38] The vestibular system is thought to be spared in the disease process, and vestibular function is found to be normal. In essence, no single audiometric configuration emerges as "the" configuration reflecting hearing loss secondary to congenital rubella. Without the obvious cause-effect suspicions raised by an epidemic, and when hearing loss is the lone clinical finding, it is difficult to recognize and identify new cases of rubella-caused hearing impairment. Historical evidence of initial vaccination followed by reinoculation, with failure to form antiagglutination titers is necessary to conclude or exclude this etiologic factor.

Once the hearing loss is confirmed, the audiological evaluations do not end. It is recommended that a close audiological surveillance continue for at least the first 3 years of life, since it is during this period that most progressions of hearing loss secondary to rubella occur. However, this is not to preclude the possibility of progressive hearing loss occurring at any other time. If parents or educators notice any change in a child's responce to sound, audiological testing should be done as soon as possible.

Furthermore, viruses have been shown to produce linguistic behavioral defects of CNS origin. If audiometric levels alone are used to judge speech and language success, important information may be missed. Therefore, continuing and diversified attempts must be made by educators to determine the hearing-impaired child's language skills.

Syphilis

Syphilis is a multi-system disease caused by infection from the spirochete, *T. pallidum*. There are often long periods of latency and latent progression of the disease as a result of the infection.

Both congenital syphilis and acquired syphilis are still recognized as causes of SNHL. Congenital syphilis is caused by intrauterine infection resulting from acquired maternal syphilis and is less responsive to antibiotic therapy than the acquired form of the disease. The incidence of maternal syphilitic infection is 0.02 per 100 pregnancies, with fetal infection occurring in 0.01 per 100 births, reflecting one of the lowest incidence rates of all chronic perinatal infections.[3]

Hearing impairment associated with congenital syphilis presents a difficult problem to the physician. Some of the complexities include the following features:

1. In up to 50% of neonatal cases, congenital syphilis may be asymptomatic.[3]
2. The routine hospital screening test for syphilis, the VDRL, shows high false-positive and -negative rates. This screen is a flocculation test that is employed universally because of its simplicity. In addition to giving a positive reaction in syphilis, it may show a positive reaction in other diseases, such as malaria, infectious hepatitis, infectious mononucleosis, and disseminated lupus erythematosus. In proven cases of late syphilis, the VDRL was found positive in 61%.[39] In contrast, the FTA-ABS is more difficult to perform and more expensive, but it is extremely sensitive. The diffuse fluorescence of syphilis must be differentiated from other conditions, such as autoimmune diseases, that produce a beaded fluorescence.[40]
3. The peak incidence of hearing loss secondary to congenital syphilis can occur at any time during the first seven decades of life. A high incidence rate occurs by the fourth decade, when neither physician nor patient may suspect the causal relationship between the congenital syphilis and the hearing loss.[41]
4. Massive penicillin therapy will not prevent or retard the progression of the hearing loss.[42]

It is reported that hearing loss will occur in 25 to 38% of patients with congenital syphilis.[43-45] The patients had had only one evaluation at the time of these studies, however, so it is possible that these percentages are low.

Syphilis and SNHL

The onset of SNHL resulting from congenital syphilis may occur in early childhood (infantile, or early form of congenital syphilis) or be delayed to adulthood (late or tardive type). Infantile SNHL usually occurs between the 8th and 12th years of life and is characterized by a sudden, bilateral, symmetrical severe hearing impairment. Vestibular signs include falling and difficulty in walking. When the onset has been delayed until adulthood, there may be only low frequency SNHL, followed by a flat asymmetrical SNHL with variation in fluctuation and progression, and commonly accompanied by episodic vertigo and tinnitus.[45] Atypical patterns of endolymphatic hydrops may occur in some cases of congenital syphilis, manifested by vertigo associated with nausea, vomiting, fluctuating hearing loss, and tinnitus. It is impossible to clinically differentiate this type of hydrops from Ménière's disease.[43]

Other variable audiological findings associated with congenital syphilis include poor discrimination scores (out of proportion to pure tone thresholds), early vestibular involvement, and rapid progression of the hearing loss.[46]

Patients with acquired syphilis tend to have more stable inner ear manifestations. Hearing loss is statistically less common in acquired syphilis.

Pathophysiology of Syphilis

The pathological changes in the inner ear secondary to syphilis, congenital or acquired, are expressed in an osteitis of all three layers of the otic capsule with inflammatory infiltration of the membranes of the cochlea and vestibular labyrinth.[43,45,47] These changes result in severe degeneration of the organ of Corti, spiral ganglion, and nerve cells along with extensive destruction of the membranous labyrinth; the resultant hearing impairment may be profound. Endolymphatic hydrops is an inner ear membrane manifestation of damage occurring from edema or fibrosis and may result in progressive degeneration of the organ of Corti and the vestibular system.

The persistence of spirochetes in the aqueous humor of the eye,[48-50] the perilymph of the ear,[51] and the tissues of the temporal bone[52] has been reported. Spirochetes remain viable despite massive therapy. It is known that penicillin does not readily cross the barrier to enter the endolymphatic fluid of the inner ear. It is, therefore, conceivable that inner ear involvement may occur after the VDRL test results have converted to negative and in the presence of a normal spinal fluid following treatment. The FTA-ABS, however, should show a positive reaction.

Diagnosis and Treatment

A VDRL should be performed on all infants suspected of having a syphilitic infection (Table 4–2). If the infant is symptomatic (50% of cases) and the FTA-ABS test is positive, therapy with large doses of aqueous penicillin G should be instituted. In the other 50% of cases, in which the infant is asymptomatic and the VDRL test results are positive, therapy should be delayed, and a concentrated effort should be made to define the nature and stage of the maternal infection (with confirmation by FTA-ABS). If it is impossible to prove that the mother with acquired syphilis has received adequate treatment, it is safer to treat the infant immediately, for these infants are at risk for congenital syphilis and its sequelae, which can be severe or even fatal. There are several physical features that can aid in the diagnosis of inner ear syphilis:

1. Physical findings such as nasal deformities (saddle nose), frontal bossing, interstitial keratitis (corneal scars), and dental manifestations (mulberry molars, Hutchinson's teeth).
2. A positive Hennebert sign (a positive fistula test in the absence of middle ear disease) is frequently present; however, it may also exist in cases of endolymphatic hydrops of Ménière's disease.[53] A positive Hennebert sign is characterized by a brief eye movement. This eye movement, which cannot be elicited by ENG, is brought about by a stimulus of negative air pressure and responds toward the eye being stimulated.
3. Perlman and Leek[54] have described a positive Tullio sign consisting of vertigo and nystagmus elicited by stimulation of the ear with a sound of loud intensity (such as with a Bárány noise box) as a finding in syphilitic inner ear disease.
4. A response to treatment is an indication of syphilitic inner ear disease. Lowered pure tone thresholds or a 10% or more improvement in discrimination scores following therapy with large doses of steroid may indicate hydrops secondary to syphilis.

Apparently, the syphilis organism, *Treponema pallidum*, has a characteristic dividing time; in early syphilis the treponeme may divide every 33 hours and in the late stages of the disease it may divide once in every 90 days. Large doses of penicillin over a period of 3 months have been proposed as the treatment of choice in the late stages of infection. Nevertheless, it is still a very difficult situation involving such decisions as a lumbar puncture (LP), a variance of protocols, and treatment for the use of antibiotics. This subject has been reviewed by Amenta et al,[55] conclud-

Table 4–2. Comparison of Serological Tests for Syphilis

Mechanism	Properties	Clinical Significance
VDRL Test for reagin in serum that reacts to nonspecific lipid antigens	Time and treatment reduce titer of reagin, may revert to seronegative. Reagin may not be fully developed in early cases (20% to 30%)	Maybe useful indicator of therapeutic responsiveness
Measurement of reactive antibodies to *Treponema pallidum*	Accuracy depends on stage of disease Reactive in 80% to 87% of untreated cases; in 90% to 99% in second stage; in 95% to 99% in latent or late stage	Specificity: positive reaction indicates disease, past or present False negative responses in infancy when antibodies have not developed
FTA-ABS Employs a sorbent that eliminates nonvirulent treponemes		

Conclusion

As a screen for neonatal syphilis, VDRL is preferred because of the simplicity of the test

Adapted from Clemis, JD.[24] Reprinted with permission.

ing that a LP is mandatory only in leutic endolymphatic hydrops patients who have neurologic signs and symptoms distinct from otologic signs and symptoms. In those patients, treatment directed toward neurosyphilis was not needed and was not cost effective.

Since syphilitic hearing impairment remains an elusive clinical diagnosis, extensive historical and physical examinations, together with appropriate laboratory testing and, in many cases, lengthy follow-ups, are necessary to validate it.

Steroids are the drugs of choice in the treatment of hearing loss secondary to congenital syphilis, although not all patients will respond to this therapy. In addition to the well-documented side effects of steroids, other problems are encountered from their use, such as an increase in hearing thresholds when medication is discontinued. There is also difficulty in determining the dose of steroids necessary to stabilize and maintain hearing threshold levels. Nevertheless, there is no choice but to institute ongoing steroid therapy for an indefinite period of time, and monthly audiograms are recommended to monitor hearing levels. After the hearing loss stabilizes, the dosage of steroid should be maintained on alternate days.

Depending on the degree of hearing loss, in all cases of fluctuating hearing or progressive hearing loss, there is an obvious hearing level at which hearing aids are beneficial. When such aids are introduced, frequent audiological evaluations of aided and unaided hearing levels are necessary until the hearing stabilizes. Unfortunately, as mentioned, not all patients with hearing loss improve with steroid treatment. However, in one study, useful hearing was maintained in 20 of 22 ears with treatment over a period of 5 to 14 years.[56] The hearing loss that does not respond will usually progress to severe-to-profound hearing impairment.

REFERENCES

1. Lyons AS, Petrucelli RJ II. In: Rowls W, ed. *Medicine: An Illustrated History.* New York, NY: Harry N Abrams; 1978:579.
2. Hinojosa R, Lindsay IR. Profound deafness: associated sensory and neural de-generation. *Arch Otolaryngol.* 1980 106:193-209.
3. Stagno S, Pass K, Alford CA. Perinatal infections and maldevelopment. *Birth Defects.* 1981;17:31-50.
4. Reynolds D, Stagno S, Stubbs G, et al. Inapparent congenital cytomegalovirus infection with elevated IgM levels: causal relation with auditory and mental deficiency. *N Engl J Med.* 1974;290:291-296.
5. Stagno S, Pass RF, Reynolds DW, et al. Comparative study diagnostic procedures for congenital CMV infection. *Pediatrics.* 1980;65:251-257.

6. Stagno S, Reynolds DW, Tsiantos A, et al. Comparative serial virologic and serologic studies of symptomatic and subclinical congenitally and natally acquired cytomegalovirus infections. *J Infect Diseases*. 1975;132:568-577.
7. Bordley JE. Hardy IMB. Laboratory and clinical observations on prenatal rubella. *Ann Otol Rhinol Laryngol*. 1969;78:917-927.
8. Pro Cit #3.
9. McGee T, Wolters C, Stein L, et al. Absence of sensorineural hearing loss in treated infants and children with congenital toxoplasmosis. *Otolaryn. Head Neck Surg*. January 1992;106(1):75-80.
10. Remington J, Demonts G. Toxoplasmosis. In: Remington J, Kelein J, eds. *Infectious Diseases of the Fetus and Newborn*. 3rd ed. Philadelphia, Pa: WB Saunders; 1990:89-195.
11. Hanshaw JB. Congenital cytomegalovirus infection: a fifteen year perspective. *J Infect Dis*. 1971;123:555-561.
12. Stern H, Tucker SM. Prospective study of cytomegalovirus infection in pregnancy. *Br Med J*. 1973; Abstract. 2:268-270.
13. Stagno S, Reynolds DW, Huang ES, et al. Congenital cytomegalovirus: occurrence in an immune population. *N Engl J Med*. 1977;296:1254-1258.
14. Weller TH. The cytomegaloviruses: ubiquitous agents with protean clinical manifestations (first of 2 parts). *N Engl J Med*. 1971;285:203-214.
15. Williamson WD, Desmond M, LaFevers N, et al. Symptomatic congenital cytomegalovirus. *Am J Dis Child*. 1982;136:902-905.
16. Pass RF, Stagno S, Meyers GJ, Alford CA Jr. Outcome of symptomatic congenital CMV infection: results of long-term longitudinal follow-up. *Pediatrics*. 1980;66:758-762.
17. Meyers E, Stool S. Cytomegalic inclusion disease of the inner ear. *Laryngoscope*. 1968;78:1904-1914.
18. Davis GL. Cytomegalovirus in the inner ear: case report and electron microscopic study. *Ann Otol Rhinol Laryngol*. 1969;78:1179-1189.
19. Davis LE, Fiber F, James CG, McLaren LC. Cytomegalovirus isolation from a human inner ear. *Ann Otol Rhinol Laryngol*. 1979;88:424-426.
20. Pappas DG. Hearing impairments and vestibular abnormalities among children with subclinical cytomegalovirus. *Ann Otol Rhinol Laryngol*. 1983;92: 552-557.
21. Stagno S, Reynolds DW, Amos CS, et al. Auditory and visual defects resulting from symptomatic and subclinical congenital cytomegaloviral and toxoplasma infections. *Pediatrics*. 1977;59:669-679.
22. Dahle AJ, McCollister FP, Hammer BA, et al. Subclinical congenital cytomegalovirus and hearing impairment. *J Speech Hear Disord*. 1974;39: 320-329.
23. Dahle AJ, McCollister FP, Stagno S, et al. Progressive hearing impairment in children with congenital cytomegalovirus infection. *J Speech Hear Disord*. 1979;44:220-229.
24. Clemis JD. Luetic labyrinthitis. *Tex Med*. 1977;73:60-65.
25. Harris JP, Woolf NK, Ryan AF, et al. Immunolologic and electrophysiologic response to cytomegalovirus inner ear infection in the guinea pig. *J Infect Dis*. 1984;150(4):523-30.

26. Gregg NM. Congenital cataract following German measles in the mother. *Trans Ophthalmol Soc Austr.* 1941;3:35-46.
27. Plotkin SA, Oski FA, Hartnett EM, et al. Some recently recognized manifestations of the rubella syndrome. *J Pediatr.* 1965;67:182-191.
28. Plotkin SA, Cochran W, Lindquist JM, et al. Congenital rubella syndrome in late infancy. *JAMA.*1967;200:105-111.
29. Alexander ER. Rubella. In: Fulginiti VA, ed. *Immunization in Clinical Practice. A Useful Guideline to Vaccines, Sera, and immune Globulins in Clinical Practice.* Philadelphia, Pa: JB Lippincott; 1982:103-111.
30. Cooper LZ, Florman AL, Ziring PR, Krugman S. Loss of rubella hemagglutination antibody in congenital rubella. *Am J Dis Child.* 1971;122:397-403.
31. Goodhill V. The nerve-deaf child: significance of Rh, maternal rubella and other etiologic factors. *Ann Otol.* 1950;59:1123-1142.
32. Schall LA, Lurie MH, Kelemen G. Embryonic hearing organs after maternal rubella. *Laryngoscope.* 1951;61:99-112.
33. Lindsay JR, Caruthers DG, Hemenway WG, Harrison S. Inner ear pathology following maternal rubella. *Ann Otol Rhinol Laryngol.* 1953;62:1201-1218.
34. Sando I, Hemenway WG, Morgan WR. Histopathology of the temporal bone in mandibulofacial dysostosis (Treacher Collins syndrome). *Trans Am Acad Ophthalmol Otolaryngol.* 1968;72:913-924.
35. Barr B, Lundstrom R. Deafness following maternal rubella. Retrospective and prospective studies. *Acta Otolaryngol.* 1961;53:413-423.
36. Borton TE, Stark EW. Audiological findings in hearing loss secondary to maternal rubella. *Pediatrics.* 1970;45:225-229.
37. Peckham CS. Clinical and laboratory study of children exposed in utero to maternal rubella. *Arch Dis Child.* 1972;47:571-577.
38. Stuckless ER, Walter GG. Students hearing impaired from the 1963-1965 rubella epidemic begin to enter college. *Volta Rev.* 1983;85:270-278.
39. Harner RE, Smith JL, Israel CW. The FTA-ABS test in late syphilis. A serological study in 1,985 cases. JAMA. 1968;203:103-106.
40. Hendershot EL. Luetic deafness. *Otolaryngol Clin North Am.* 1978;11:43-47.
41. Steckelberg JM, McDonald TJ. Otologic involvement in late syphilis. *Laryngoscope.* 1984;94:753-757.
42. Patterson ME. Congenital luetic hearing impairment. *Arch Otolaryngol.* 1968;878:70-74.
43. Karmody CS, Schuknecht HF. Deafness in congenital syphilis. *Arch Otolaryngol.* 1966;83:44-53.
44. Dalsgaard-Nielsen E. Correlation between syphilitic interstitial keratitis and deafness. *Acta Ophthalmol.* 1938;16:635-646.
45. Schuknecht HF. *Pathology of the Ear.* Cambridge, Ma: Harvard University Press; 1974:263.
46. Nadol JB Jr. Hearing loss of acquired syphilis: diagnosis confirmed by incudectomy. *Laryngoscope.* 1975;85:1888-1897.
47. Goodhill V. Syphilis of the ear. A histopathological study. *Ann Otol Rhinol Laryngol.* 1939;48:676-706.

48. Christman EH, Hamilton RW, Heaton CL, Hoffmeyer IM. Intraocular treponemes. *Arch Ophthalmol.* 1968;80:303-307.
49. Goldman JN, Girard KF. Intraocular treponemes in treated congenital syphilis. *Arch Ophthalmol.* 1967;78:47-50.
50. Smith JL, Israel CW, McCrary JA, Harmer RE. Recovery of Treponema pallidum from aqueous humor removed at cataract surgery in man by passive transfer to rabbit testis. *Am J Ophthalmol.* 1968;65:242-247.
51. Wiet RJ, Milko DA. Isolation of the spirochetes in the perilymph despite prior antisyphilitic therapy. *Arch Otolaryngol.* 1975;101:104-106.
52. Mack LW, Smith JL, Walter EK, et al. Temporal bone treponemes. *Arch Otolarygol.* 1969;90:11-14.
53. Nadol JB. Positive "fistula sign" with an intact tympanic membane. Clinical report of three cases and histopathological description of vestibulofibrosis as the probably cause. *Arch Otolaryngol.* 1974;100:273-278.
54. Perlman HB, Leek JH. Late congenital syphilis of the ear. *Laryngoscope.* 1952;62:1175-1196.
55. Amenta C, Dayal V, Flaherty J, Weil R. Leutic endolymphatic hydrops: diagnosis and treatment. *Amer J Otol.* November 1992;13(No.6):516-524.
56. Adams DA, Kerr AG, Smyth GDC, Cinnamond MJ. Congenital syphilitic deafness. A further review. *J Laryngol Otol.* 1983;97:399-404.

5

Acquired Hearing Loss Due to Other Infections and Causes

> *You can . . . never foretell what any one man will do, but you can say with precision what an average number will be up to. Individuals vary, but percentages remain constant.*
>
> The Sign of Four
> *Sherlock Holmes*

SEROUS OTITIS MEDIA

The hearing loss resulting from serous otitis media (SOM) (Fig 5–1) is most commonly conductive in nature. However, the impact SOM has on preexisting SNHL is so great that guidelines for treatment are needed.

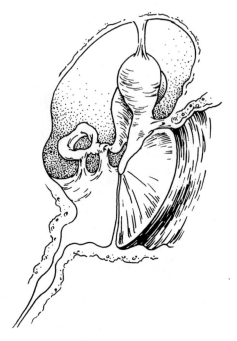

Fig 5-1.— Middle ear cavity with fluid.

For normal hearing patients there are other than medical reasons for concern when SOM persists because of a lack of vigorous treatment, continuous drainage, the failure of ventilation tubes to provide aeration of the tympanic cavity, or lingering negative pressure without evidence of middle ear effusion. In a significant number of such cases, the associated "temporary" hearing loss may last for periods of months to years, and the children so affected have been found to suffer language delays.[1,2] To prevent this possibility, implementation of speech and language evaluation, amplification, and consideration of medical or surgical intervention, or both, should be initiated in the early stages of this disease process.

Definition and Classifications

Acute inflammation of the middle ear (acute otitis media) is also known as suppurative, purulent, or bacterial otitis media, and is a frequent cause of conductive hearing loss, most often in the range of 15 to 40 dB.

Acute otitis media probably accompanies every viral upper respiratory infection (URI). The mucosa of the pharynx is continuous with the mucosa of the eustachian tube and middle ear; therefore, a mucositis of the nasal, pharyngeal, paranasal, or sinus membranes will extend into the eustachian tube to produce a tubotympanitis. Most URIs are transitory and the tubotympanitis subsides without complication. In some cases, however, a secondary or primary bacterial infection occurs that causes an acute otitis media. In these cases, SOM will most commonly develop, which is sometimes referred to as secretory otitis, nonsuppurative otitis, mucoid otitis, or otitis media with effusion. During episodes of suppurative (infected) otitis media or serous (noninfected) otitis media, fluid accumulates in the middle ear and the tympanic membrane may rupture spontaneously. In chronic cases, the most common method of management is myringotomy with the insertion of a ventilation tube. In other patients, a chronic otitis media (more commonly called suppurative or purulent otitis media) may develop. In this stage of ear disease, there is a chronic inflammation of the middle ear and mastoid. Spontaneous rupture of the tympanic membrane ensues, a central perforation develops, and a discharge (otorrhea) is present.

Incidence

SOM occurs in people of all ages but is seen predominantly in children. The peak incidence occurs in the 6- to 24-month age group, declining in frequency to age 7 years, after which it becomes even less common.[3]

The incidence of recurrent, chronic, or severe SOM is widespread among certain racial groups, such as Eskimos and American Indians; blacks, on the other hand, have a lower incidence rate than whites.[4] This difference in frequency among races reflects anatomical and genetic factors; however, the role of socioeconomic conditions has not been delineated.

A number of conditions predispose infants and children to persistent SOM and negative pressure (Table 5–1). These include cleft palate and cleft uvula (up to 70%),[5] immune deficiency states (agammaglobulinemia, hypogammaglobulinemia),[6] and syndromes (Down's syndrome, 36%[7-9]; mucopolysaccharidosis; Apert's syndrome; and so forth). Other presumptive reasons for a predisposition to SOM include a history of family members with speech-language or SOM problems, or both. A genetic predisposition to middle ear infection is suggested by the fact that multiple instances of SOM occur in some families.[10] Children who have an isolated bout or recurrent episodes of SOM are more likely to have sib-

Table 5–1. Conditions Associated With High Risk for Otitis Media With Effusion

Cleft palate or cleft uvula

Immunity deficiency

Syndromic children

Preexisting SNHL or negative pressure

History of family member(s) with speech-language or serous otitis media problems

lings with a history of significant middle ear infections than are children who have had no episodes of SOM. Consequently, information regarding older, normally hearing siblings who have had SOM, behavioral problems, or speech or language development difficulties is of significance in such cases.

Most of the foregoing categories were described by Downs,[5] who also includes in her list those children who have their first bout of SOM prior to age 18 months. However, it is difficult to ascertain the age at which SOM might have the greatest effect on speech and language development. Studies of language development in children indicate that there are distinct changes in the linguistic abilities of children throughout their developmental period of birth to 8 years of age.[11] Persistent SOM with hearing deprivation would be more detrimental at an age of less than 18 months for two different reasons. One reason is that birth to 1 year of age is the period in which the ability to discriminate between speech sounds of lengthier contexts is developing. The second reason for the detrimental affect of SOM occurring prior to age 18 months, when discrimination of second syllable consonant contrasts is learned (Examples: renew-review; inside-insight), is that those children who have this experience tend to have recurrences over an extended period of time and are, therefore, said to be "otitis prone," whereas children who have their first episode of SOM after age 18 months do not have such extended histories.[12]

Complications From Chronic Otitis Media

In a study of 123 human temporal bones from persons affected by chronic otitis media, Meyerhoff and coworkers[13] identified osteitis (in 90% of all specimens), fibrosis of the subepithelial space (76%), granulation tissue

(69%), tympanosclerosis (28%), cholesteatoma (15%), and cholesterol granuloma (13%). This same study showed a relatively low incidence of tympanic membrane perforation (19.5%).

Histological studies of both human and animal temporal bones have shown varying degrees of pathological involvement of the round window and scala tympani of the basal turn adjacent to the round window membrane.[14] Findings included abnormal or missing hair cells in the basal turn.

Endolymphatic hydrops associated with otitis media has been identified both clinically and histologically[15] in a study of 560 human temporal bones in which 109 demonstrated hydrops and 194 showed otitis media. Both otitis media and hydrops coexisted in 75 cases.

Because of the proximity of the CNS to the middle ear, life-threatening complications of otitis media, although rare, still exist. These include labyrinthitis, coalescent mastoiditis, petrositis, meningitis, lateral sinus thrombophlebitis, otic hydrocephalus, and intracranial abscesses. The role of otitis media in meningitis is thought to be one of coexistence. Most cases of meningitis are believed to be due to URIs causing hematogenous spread to the meninges and then to the inner ear.

Sequelae of otitis media are more common and should be differentiated from complications.[3] These sequelae usually include those conditions resulting in structural damage to the middle ear itself and leading to physiological changes of the hearing mechanism. Included in this group are atrophic changes of the tympanic membrane and epithelial layers of the middle ear mucosa, osteitis with erosion of the ossicular chain (particularly the long process of the incus), tympanosclerosis, formation of granulation tissue, cholesteatoma, and cholesterol granuloma. These sequelae may even occur with the best medical treatment, and their appearance requires surgical intervention.

Preexisting Sensorineural Hearing Loss and Negative Pressure

Infants and young children with SNHL are as prone to experience episodes of otitis media with effusion as a comparable group of normal hearing population. Indeed, considering the etiology of SNHL with its high-risk factors, including cranial facial anomalies, then these children with SNHL may be at an increased risk for otitis media with effusion.[16]

Negative middle ear pressure can cause a significant decrease in hearing, especially in the child with a preexisting SNHL. Subjective signs of diminished performance in hearing and learning have been observed by educators and parents (observation by ECHO Foundation). Hearing thresholds decrease in the low and high frequencies as they may in normally hearing children with negative pressure.

In a study of 44 normally hearing children, middle ear pressure of –150 mm to –250 mm of water pressure (mm H_2O) occurs in 25 to 55% at different times of the year, and conductive hearing losses of 10 to 20 decibels (dB) were found in seven of these children.[17] Middle ear pathology should be considered when the pressure is greater than –150 mm H_2O, when a flat audiogram is evident, or when pure tone screening levels are greater than 20 dB at 500 to 4000 Hz. Although negative middle ear pressure may affect the hearing acuity of normally hearing children, the criteria for medical or surgical intervention have not been established because speech frequencies are not affected.[18] However, a loss of 10 dB or more in a child who is hearing-impaired using amplification is obviously detrimental and, should medical treatment not alleviate the negative pressure, surgical intervention with ventilation tubes must be carried out no later than 6 weeks after the hearing decrease is determined.

A group of 25 patients with SNHL and negative pressure were closely monitored by the author. In two of these patients, increased thresholds were observed with negative pressure as low as –50 mm H_2O. Increased hearing thresholds (15 dB or more) were observed for most, or all, frequencies even in the presence of negative middle ear pressure. This superimposed hearing loss further encroaches on the ability to listen (hearing) and slows the process of speech and language acquisition. Consider a child who is identified as having hearing impairment at age 12 months, with pure tone threshold levels of 70 dB. Aided hearing response is in Ling and Ling's "speech banana"[19] for most frequencies. However, the child's learning ability may be adversely affected because the negative middle ear pressure increases the threshold of hearing. The urgency of relieving this negative pressure, which has been known to persist or recur for a year, becomes obvious when we consider that this child was 1 year old when the hearing loss was identified, and the child consequently was already a year behind normally hearing peers in speech and language skills. At this important stage in development, any obstacle to such a child's acquisition of these skills could be crucial to the youngster's progress. It is recommended that an impedance audiometer be used to examine for middle ear pressure prior to each therapy session for all children in a program for those with hearing impairment, especially when amplification with hearing aids is employed. Ventilation tubes are indicated if negative middle ear pressure (–150 mm H_2O or greater) persists continuously for 6 weeks. This is aggressive treatment, but of what value is 6 weeks of therapy sessions with a 15 dB decrease superimposed on a moderate to profound hearing loss?

Organism and Drug-Related Factors

Table 5–2 lists a sample of the published studies related to the association between infectious agents and instances of SOM. This compilation has identified *Streptococcus pneumoniae, Haemophilus influenzae*, and *Moraxella catarrhalis* as the most frequent etiological agents present, with approximately 15% of the cultures of the middle ear being sterile.

Effective treatment of pneumococci and *H. influenzae* infections is provided today by many microbial agents such as ampicillin and amoxicillin, the combination of erythromycin and sulfonamides and, more recently, a combination of trimethoprim and sulfamethoxazole. There is no evidence for therapeutic efficacy of systemic antihistamines and decongestants in the absence of nasal allergy.[23]

Much of the decrease in complications of otitis media must be attributed to the widespread use of antibiotics. Unfortunately, however, antibi-

Table 5–2. Incidence of Infectious Agents in Acute Serous Otitis Media

Infectious Agents	Incidence
Haemophilus influenzae	23%; most common from birth to 2 years, but significant throughout childhood [20]
Diplococcus pneumoniae	35%[20]
Moraxella catarrhalis	14%[20]
Group A beta hemolytic streptococcus	3%[20]
Staphylococcus aureus	Infrequent[20]
Gram-negative bacilli	Common in newborn ICU nursery (20–30%)[21,22]
Viruses	Isolated in 4.4% of 663 patients; respiratory syncytial and influenza viruses most frequent,[21] maybe as common as 33%
Mycoplasma pneumoniae	Have been difficult to isolate from middle ear effusion[12]
Chlamydia trachomatis	In some 6 months or younger

otic therapy has not had a favorable influence on the outcome of the disease process in some cases of otitis media. It is important that the clinician be aware of the following reasons for this:

1. Although viruses are only rarely recovered from middle ear effusions,[20,21] the epidemiological association of antecedent or concurrent viral infections is strong.[24]
2. An increased number of organisms have become resistant to ampicillin, especially the beta-lactamase producing *Haemophilus influenzae*.[25]
3. Hitherto unidentified organisms with the potential of causing suppurative otitis media, such as *Moaxella*[26] and anaerobic bacteria[27] have been of increasing prominence.

Pathogenesis

It is commonly agreed that infection is the basic etiological factor in SOM although, traditionally, specific disorders of the eustachian tube (such as the inability to ventilate the middle ear) have been considered to be the real culprit. There are indications that persistent SOM is a local immune response dependent on repeated acute middle ear infections or the result of antigens of microorganisms migrating from the nasopharynx. Patients with or without an immune deficiency may be susceptible to these persistent stimuli. Nonetheless, the role of the eustachian tube should not be discounted. Numerous studies[28-30] show variability of eustachian tube function. In normal children, these studies indicate that the younger the patient, the poorer the eustachian tube function. Another predisposing factor for otitis media effusion, an allergic pathogenesis, has been advocated, but not confirmed. Many investigators have marked the relationship between allergy and otitis media effusion, but the definite allergic mechanisms by which antigen affects the eustachian tube and tympanic cavity are not clear. One function seems definite, that the eustachian tube protects the middle ear from antigenic invasion from the nasopharynx.

Recent advances in immunology and biochemistry of the middle ear cavity have established that the inflamed mucosa has many attributes of an immune response; however, the evidence regarding this hypothesis is mixed. Though secretory IgA is found in middle ear effusions, IgG is considered the main defense mechanism in the middle ear against bacterial infection, and IgG antibodies may be the key factor in production of the secondary response that produces middle ear effusion.[31] Support for such a chain of events is shown by various investigators, such as Mogi[32] who injected protein antigen into the tympanic cavity of immunized animals and produced effusion; and Pelton et al[33] who observed IgG_2 subclass in children with recurrent acute otitis media compared with patients free from middle ear disease. This secretory immune response has been initiated by a series of biological events in which a chain of enzymatic reactions, mediated by complement, is set in motion. It involves complement activation through a series of interacting plasma proteins, which results in increased vascular permeability, accumulation of leukocytes, enhanced phagocytosis, cell lysis, and destruction of the invasive organisms. A continuous release of enzymes promotes these activities, resulting in the release of substrates; this could explain the persistence of middle ear effusion without the presence of bacteria or the continuous drainage through a ventilation tube that occurs in some patients.

In essence, when the various times of onset of otitis media effusion are placed in chronological order based on the recent literature, the following conclusions are reached:

1. Bacteria (most commonly *Streptococcus pneumoniae* and *Haemophilus influenzae*) are harbored in the nasopharynx. Inflammation initiates eustachian tube obstruction and middle ear edema or middle ear edema without eustachian tube obstruction. In such situations, bacteria is cultured from the middle ear.[34-36]
2. Effusion occurs in the middle ear of children harboring pharyngeal bacteria, the microbes providing the antigen. Even with inactive bacteria, as shown in animal studies, the endotoxin may provide the antigen.[37,38]
3. Chronicity of effusion, in spite of antibiotic therapy, may be due to resistant strains of bacteria, prolonged eustachian tube obstruction, recurrence of nasopharyngeal infection, or other causes.

Studies showing any real efficacy of adenoidectomy in alleviating middle ear effusion do not fully support the surgical procedure.[39-41] Browning and Gatehouse's recent investigation has indicated that, in cases of otitis media with effusion, benefits result from the removal of the involved adenoid tissue and insertion of ventilation tubes gave better hearing results after 6 months than did adenoidectomy alone, or tubes alone.[42] Although evidence of benefit from early adenoid removal is lacking, the purpose of such removal is to eliminate the harboring of bacteria and viruses. The study of Pillsbury and coworkers shows a reduction in the incidence of pathogenic organisms following adenoidectomy.[43]

The role of nasal allergy is not clearly defined. However, when antigens are introduced into the eustachian tube, a topical reaction occurs in the middle ear. Medications, according to studies,[44] have been shown to prevent eustachian tube obstruction and provide relief of symptoms. At this point, the number of subjects studied is small, but research is continuing.

Clinically, it is difficult to determine the biochemical and immuno-logical characteristics of middle ear effusions without sophisticated laboratory investigations; such studies have been under way.[45]

Benefits of Ventilation Tubes

The clear advantages of ventilation tubes include the elimination of conductive hearing loss, reduction in the recurrence of acute otitis media, and avoidance of linguistic, social, and cognitive developmental delays. Ventilation tubes may have no direct influence on the underlying disease, but this remains uncertain and, if the SOM is the result of an immune response, adequate ventilation and removal of fluid may well lead to a permanent resolution. The question is not one of the validity of this procedure, but when it is indicated.[46]

Each case is a unique situation and many factors (such as the patient's age, age at onset of symptoms, duration of symptoms, intensity of treatment, structural changes of the tympanic membrane, delay in speech and language development), are involved in decision making (Table 5–3).

Other indications for tubes include chronic otitis media with history of more than one perforation, or when a separate complication is present, such as facial paralysis, presence of eustachian tube dysfunction causing hearing loss of 30 dB or more air-bone gap, otalgia, vertigo, or tinnitus. Other indications for tubes are some isolated cases of tympanoplasty that are aggravated by eustachian tube dysfunction.

The physical examination is as important as the historical data. Tympanometry cannot be relied on, as it can identify, but not necessarily quantify, structural damage to the tympanic membrane. The appearance

---

Table 5–3. Indications for Placement of Ventilation Tubes

- Continuous effusion for 3 months or longer

- Frequent (plus 4) episodes of otitis media lasting 3 weeks or more each

- Structural changes in the tympanic membrane, such as a retraction pocket, atrophy, retraction

- Chronic otitis media with history of more than one perforation

- Concurrent SNHL and persistent negative middle ear pressure

---

of the tympanic membrane is the most important aspect of the physical examination and can, in many instances, indicate whether or not a tympanotomy with insertion of a ventilation tube is necessary. When evaluating the status of the tympanic membrane and tympanum, the examiner should be observant for the following possibilities:

1. The presence of deep yellow-orange fluid and a chalky appearance of the handle of the malleus associated with a prominent neck of the malleus, which indicates retraction of the tympanic membrane or chronicity of the SOM.
2. The appearance of localized retraction areas, usually found in the posterior-superior portion of the drumhead, where the incus and its connection to the stapes may become very obvious, indicating chronic eustachian tube obstruction. Other areas where localized retraction pockets may be identified are in the pars flaccida and in the inferior or anterior portions of the drumhead.
3. Changes in the tympanic membrane suggesting localized or generalized atrophy, which usually occurs with retraction (this should encourage early intervention with ventilation tubes).
4. The presence of a light-colored fluid that is not too obvious but, when coexisting with immobility of the tympanic membrane, may indicate chronicity of the SOM. Again, tympanometry is no substitute for a pneumatic otoscopic examination with special sealed speculae through which the physician is able to observe the structural changes and mobility of the tympanic membrane.
5. Hearing levels of 35 dB or greater, which may indicate chronicity of middle ear fluid.
6. Evidence (or history) of persistent rupturing of the tympanic membranes.
7. Other abnormalities of the drumhead, such as fluid with air bubbles, bright-colored fluid with good mobility of the tympanic membranes, or blue or black fluid (indicating middle ear bleeding) may not require tympanotomies with ventilation tubes; patients with such abnormalities may be monitored.

Again, each case is unique and the course of intervention may be different for each patient. Certainly, a patient with a red, bulging drumhead who is febrile and irritable should have an immediate myringotomy.

Tympanotomy without ventilation tubes has not been so efficacious in the prevention of recurrent disease or the alleviation of a conductive hearing loss.[47]

Surgical Management

The ventilation tube establishes aeration of the tympanic cavity for patients with chronic SOM. Preferably, a small incision is made by a small, sharp knife into the anterior middle portion of the tympanic membrane. Most acoustic energy is conveyed by the posterior one half of the tympanic membrane, and tube placement in this area may cause a mild conductive hearing loss. Special consideration is given to controlling even minute bleeding that might later dry and form a crust that may block the ventilation tube or hinder mobility of the tympanic membrane. The middle ear fluid is evacuated as completely as possible. A short (button variety) tube is preferred, especially in the child wearing hearing aids. Some excessively long tubes are manipulated with earmold casting and, in addition, long tubes have a tendency to become blocked with cerumen as the earmold builds up and pushes the cerumen toward the tympanic membrane. The duration of a functioning ventilation tube may depend on individual characteristics of the tube, such as the diameter, size of the medial flange, the number of flanges inserted[48] (Fig 5–2), or placement in the anterior portion of the tympanic membrane (where epithelial migration is minimal). With larger medial flanges, there may be greater probability of a permanent perforation. Care must be taken to avoid touching the tube to the mucosa of the middle ear when placing the ventilation tube deep into the tympanic cavity. Seepage of serous discharge and formation of granulation tissue from contact of the tube with the mucosa may block the tube or cause recurrent inflammation. In such a situation, the ventilation tube should be removed.

Intubation of the tympanic membrane as a treatment for chronic SOM has no therapeutic effect on the malfunctioning eustachian tube. Clinically, in most cases, it reduces the incidence of effusion of the middle ear. It also reduces the incidence and severity of pathological changes in the subepithelial space of the middle ear.[49]

Type of Tube Employed

The type of tube employed varies tremendously with the surgeon. The most commonly used tube is the double phalange tube with 1 mm of tubing between the phalanges. This tube typically stays in approximately 1 year, aerates well, and functions well. Long tubes with one phalange that are inserted into the middle ear are easier to employ, but have a greater risk of obstruction of the lumen from secretions from the middle ear. Tubes with a small lumen tend to obstruct more easily. Tubes with larger lumens tend to have a greater opportunity to cause a permanent perforation.

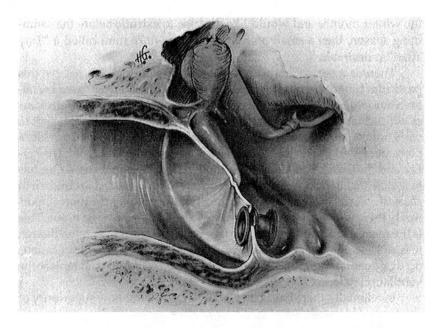

Fig 5-2.—Triflange tube showing 1.5 mm (2 flange) insertion of tube into tympanic cavity. Average duration time for this tube, so placed, is 18 months; one flange in tympanum averages 12 months with 1 mm tube insertion or 6 months with 0.5 mm insertion. From DG Pappas.[48] Reprinted with permission.

The author utilizes five different types of tubes, depending on the uniqueness of the situation. The most common tube routinely used by the author is shaped like an hourglass, has two phalanges that are not very prominent, and has a sloping 1 mm of tubing that is shaped like a saddle. There is less crusting with such a tube if the tube remains intact for any length of time. It remains intact for 9-12 months. If the patient's situation requires a tube for a greater length of time, for instance in a case that is known to extrude tubes very easily, then a triphalange tube is employed. This is a tube that is 1.5 mm in length and has three phalanges. Two phalanges are inserted into the tympanum. Such a tube will stay intact for approximately 18 months. In a patient with atelectasis, who has had multiple tubes, has atrophy, or does not maintain a tube well, a titanium large bore tube (.045 cm) is used. In these cases, it may be an advantage to have a perforation to aerate the ear. If a tube is desired for a short period of time (4-6 months) for a tympanoplasty case, or in a patient who needs it just for the winter months and would like the tube to extrude before the swimming season, then a small bore titanium tube (0.76 mm) called a "Tiny Titan" is desirable.

There is a permanent tube in the armamentarium. We reserve this particular tube for adults. Typically, permanent tubes are not used in children since the incidence of otitis media, effusion, and atelectasis decreases with advancing age. There is a tendency for many otolaryngologists to use a "more permanent tube" to try to stay in longer, and even to create a permanent perforation, which is, of course, sometimes desirable. The Per-Lee and the Goode T tubes have been utilized for these purposes. One has to realize that the more of a permanent effect that is needed in children in cases of atelectasis (atrophy of the tympanic membrane), the more opportunity there is for developing crust, blockage, and granulation tissue. This is the main reason that I prefer the large bore titanium tube, even though it is not always free of such complications. When such complications occur, a general anesthetic usually must be used to cleanse and replace the ventilation tube.

Incidentally, there has been no data available to show superiority of one type of biomedical material over another.

Complications With Ventilation Tubes

No surgical treatment is without the possibility of complications. The incidence of otorrhea following the insertion of ventilation tubes has been reported in the literature to vary from 5% to 21%.[50,51] Typically, otorrhea following ventilation tube insertion is a short-term problem. Statistics may differ according to the patient's environment and host defense, underlying cause (eg, cleft palate, immune deficiency, ciliary abnormality), type of ventilation tube used, and site of insertion in the tympanic membrane and preexisting bacteria in the effusion. Although a ventilation tube, plastic or metal, is capable of initiating the formation of granulation tissue according to J Pappas (personal communication), granuloma formation may be more prevalent when the tube chosen is made of Silastic or when a flange is positioned so that it touches the mucosa of the tympanum. The possibility that an outer flange, lying against the tympanic membrane, might instigate crust and subsequent granulation tissue formation has been suggested by Armstrong and Armstrong.[52] However, the most probable cause of persistent or intermittent drainage is the initial disease process itself. Once drainage through a ventilation tube starts (or persists), the following principles are applied:

1. When the drainage is initiated by the presence of URI, the most common cause of a nasopharyngeal infection is *H. influenzae* or *S. pneumoniae*,[53] and antibiotics are the treatments of choice.

2. Try to avoid ototoxic otic drops such as neomycin (in Cortisporin, Colymycin S, Otobiotic, Neodecadron) and gentamycin (Garamycin). Animal studies have shown that the application of these otic drops to the external ear canal with patent tympanostomy tubes may result in high frequency impairment and cochlear hair cell loss.[54] There are theories, however, as to why there is little documented ototoxicity in humans with the widespread use of aminoglycoside eardrops. It may be argued that in humans, these topical preparations may never diffuse through the round window membrane, since they are predominantly used during periods of inflammatory edema. Another reason that the drug may not absorb into the inner ear may be due to the oblique orientation of the human round window, or poor penetration through the oblique human round window.

   Most otolaryngologists use ototopical preparations in the presence of a perforation, especially one that is draining, in the presence of drainage through a ventilation tube, and in the presence of a tympanomastoid cavity. There seem to have been no reports of known irreversible inner ear damage, although one report has indicated that 3.4% of its respondents had witnessed irreversible inner ear damage, unquestionably related to the ototopicals.[55] However, the potential risk of hearing impairment contraindicates the use of these medications in most cases, especially for a child with a preexisting SNHL. One should try to be very selective in the use or need of these otic medications, and the physician should be communicative enough to warn the patient to cease the medication once the drainage has subsided.[56] An otic preparation containing Cefmenoxine was tested by applying it to the round window membrane of the chinchilla by Ikeda et al.[57] The long-term cochleotoxicity was evaluated by electrocochleography. These animals were also treated with Cortisporin and the findings indicate that the Cephalosporin was nontoxic compared with Cortisporin, thus adding a nontoxic otic drop to one's armamentarium.

3. Also to be avoided is the use of otic drops with acid carriers, but only because these preparations are painful when applied to the middle ear mucosa. Excluding the otic preparations containing neomycin and gentamycin, eardrops containing acid carriers include chloramphenicol (Chloromycetin), polymyxin B (Pyocidin), and acetic acid (Vosol). Vasocidin, an ophthalmic drug containing sulfacetamide sodium but no acid carrier, is one alternative preparation.

Unfortunately, a common contaminant in cases of otorrhea spread by means of tympanostomy tubes is *Pseudomonas aeruginosa*. Thorough cleansing of the ear canal followed by insufflation of a powder mixture of chloromycetin, sulfadiazine, and amphotericin (Fungizone) (CSF powder)[58] into the ear once or twice daily has proved to be effective in the control of this type of otorrhea. When the foregoing treatment cannot be accomplished at home, daily visits to the office are necessary.

Of all medical treatments that have been advocated, the importance of mechanical cleansing of cerumen and infectious debris from the ear canal and bacterial culture of the material is not to be overlooked. Should the drainage be copious, or should the ear canal be obstructed with cerumen or debris, the medication will not penetrate the lumen of the ventilation tube or middle ear mucosa. In some cases, daily cleansing may be necessary.

Failure of the site of perforation to heal after extrusion of a ventilation tube is reported to occur in 1.8% of cases, but increases significantly in the use of long stay tubes (as Goode type).[59] There is a possible common underlying factor in cases of nonclosure of the tympanotomy site and persistent eustachian tube obstruction. Also reported is that 1.7% of the cases have cholesteatoma formation,[60] although this small figure outweighs the benefits of intubation in preventing cholesteatoma by retraction.

Another physical finding in children with middle ear effusion is tympanosclerosis. It has been reported that ears with serous fluid are more likely to develop tympanosclerosis than ears with other types of effusion.[61] Furthermore, an antigen-antibody reaction process has been implicated as the cause of tympanosclerosis.[62] The role of ventilation tubes in the formation of tympanosclerosis, should there be one, has not been elucidated.

When To Remove a Ventilation Tube

There are two scenarios that present in this type of situation. The first situation is the patient who has had ventilation tubes for 3-4 years and has had no symptoms during this time, and has no symptoms at the present time. Should these ventilation tubes be removed? If the tubes have been present for 3 years, I would say give it another year. If it has been in place for 4 years, it is my preference, in an asymptomatic patient, to remove the tubes if there is a very negative history with regard to URIs, no evidence of drainage through the ventilation tubes, especially in the preceding year, and physical examination of the tympanic membranes that shows no evidence of atrophy or other physical changes that may indicate chronic inflammation.

The second scenario is where a ventilation tube is typically in one ear, and there is negative pressure in the other ear. In this case, I would leave this tube in indefinitely, and try to monitor the child at least every 4 months. If there is no evidence of negative pressure in the ear without the tube for 4 months, then I would remove the ventilation tube.

Another example is a child who has a ventilation tube intact, it has been so for 2 or more years, and there is granulation tissue, polyp formation, drainage, the patient has typically been on antibiotics for 6 weeks or more, and local treatment has been employed. In such a case, the tube is symptomatic and should be removed.

A consideration that should be taken is the season of the year and ensuing swimming months. Indeed, one would tend not to remove a long-term ventilation tube in autumn, since the most common season for URIs is the winter months. For further discussion on this subject, one is referred to Bluestone and Klein, *Otitis Media in Infants and Children*, 2nd Edition, Saunders, 1995, pages 212-213.

Protection From Water When Tubes Are in Place

It is very difficult for water, especially while bathing, to get through the small lumen of a ventilation tube; the surface tension of the water probably prevents the fluid from going through the tube. Usually, water will get through when one puts his or her head under water for any length of time. For this reason, it is best to try and protect the ear when tubes are in place. If no water plugs or sound plugs are available, then cotton or lamb's wool "messed" with vaseline or petroleum jelly applied to the concha will suffice. Soft plugs, preferably with large phalanges of different sizes pressed into the external auditory canal will seal water from the ear canal. It is unnecessary to use more expensive, custom-made molds for the purpose of swimming or bathing. There are a wide variety of sound plugs on the market that probably are better suited for preventing water from getting into the ear canal.

One must use caution to try to get a well-fitting, preferably phalange-type ear plug for swimming deeply under water. One must have a plug that will not easily dislodge from the ear canal, as contamination of the middle ear will certainly result.

Technique of Closure of Posttympanotomy Perforation

In those few cases in which extrusion of a tympanotomy tube results in a perforation of the drumhead, an extensive operation for closure is not necessary. Timing of the closure is, however, critical. Function of the eustachian tube should be evaluated and, although this cannot be done definitively in any one manner, the following possibilities or factors should be considered:

1. Absence of ear infections or negative pressure, especially in the opposite ear.
2. Degree of dampness in the perforated ear: preferably a dry ear for 1 year.
3. Absence of scarring or retraction with adhesions or atrophy of the remainder of the drumhead. When such conditions exist, it may be better to leave the perforation for permanent aeration of the middle ear or prepare for a tympanoplasty at a later date (after the age of 8 years) so that the ossicular chain may be evaluated.
4. Testing eustachian tube function subjectively by the use of such methods as the Politzer maneuver, or objectively by measuring the pressure required to open the tube through the tympanic membrane perforation by impedance methods.
5. Degree of hearing loss: Perforations that persist following ventilation tube extrusion typically cause little or no hearing loss. In this situation, surgery should be postponed until the patient is older (10 years of age) to ensure optimum function of the eustachian tube. It is advisable to correct the perforation in patients with a bilateral hearing loss of greater than 15 dB in the higher speech frequencies (4000 Hz) to give optimum hearing for speech and language development.

The procedure described by Derlacki[63] using trichloroacetic acid and cotton soaked with U-Mol* may be accomplished in the office without anesthesia to close the perforation in older pediatric patients; younger children require anesthesia. In a different procedure (Fig 5–3), a fat graft is taken from the lobule of the ear and placed as an underlay on the inner surface of the perforation. In this method, three preparations are made before the graft is applied: (1) the squamous epithelium on the edge of the perforation is removed with a No. 59 eye blade Beaver knife, (2) Gelfoam is packed from the middle wall of the tympanum to the surface of the tympanic membrane and the perforation, and (3) the clump of fat is pressed in the Gelfoam presser to form a flat membrane. The fat membrane is then carefully tucked underneath the edges of the perforation throughout its circumference. For support, a large, flattened square of Gelfoam is placed externally to cover the graft and edges of the tympanic membrane. On postoperative follow-ups, the Gelfoam is left untouched,

*Eucalyptol, methyl salicylate, thymol, menthol, oil of orange, sodium borate, boric acid, alcohol, and saffarin-O in distilled water.

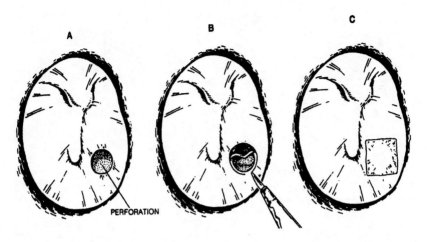

Fig 5-3.—Technique for closure of a perforation of the tympanic membrane. A, that results from ventilation tube. B, Perforation edge removal with No. 59 Beaver blade. C, Underlying fat graft with flattened square of Gelfoam overlying the graft for support.

and some months later the graft becomes visible. Closure occurs in over 90% of the cases in which this technique is applied.

CONGENITAL CHOLESTEATOMA

Although cholesteatomas do not usually cause SNHL, this topic is included in this section because of the differential diagnoses that occur in some cases of SOM. A congenital cholesteatoma is found most commonly between birth and 5 years of age. It is important to diagnose this condition promptly, as a delay presents a threat to the ossicular chain, which will be disrupted either by the disease itself or by the more aggressive surgery that is mandated by its continuation.

Congenital cholesteatomas are typically located in the anterior middle or superior portion of the pars tensa of the tympanic membrane. On examination of the ear, they are seen as a white, round, or oval mass on the mucous membrane of the middle ear cavity. They also appear to extend deep, beyond the tympanic membrane, in contrast to tympanosclerosis, in which the lesion is located within the drumhead (Fig 5–4, A).

The diagnosis of a congenital cholesteatoma can be made only by otoscopic examination, since audiometry usually reveals the hearing ability to be within normal range, and tympanometry is unreliable

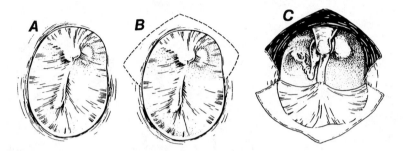

Fig 5-4.—Approach for removal of small congenital cholesteatoma. A, Typical site of congenital cholesteatoma. B, Incision in superior external auditory canal. C, Exposure of tympanum with flap extended interiorly.

because there is no attachment of the mass to the tympanic membrane. All physicians, and especially pediatricians, should examine their patients' ears for the presence of a congenital cholesteatoma, although this lesion is rare (an educated guess would be 1 in 2000 patients).

The best approach for surgical removal of a congenital cholesteatoma (Fig 5-4) following general anesthesia and local infiltration of lidocaine (Xylocaine) into the vascular strip, is a wide superior tympanotomy flap. The flap and the canal skin, pars flaccida, a portion of the pars tensa (down to its attachment to the umbo) are elevated downward (Fig 5-4, B and C).

Then the cholesteatoma is usually well-exposed. Every attempt should be made to remove the mass in toto as sectional removal increases the chances of leaving some matrix. A microscopic mirror is an essential tool in examining the underparts of the malleus for any residue of the cholesteatoma. Disarticulation of the ossicular chain (removal of the incus, then the head of the malleus) is necessary when the growth or mass extends into the attic area. When the cholesteatoma is extensive, reexamination by tympanotomy will be required approximately 1 year following surgery. In those cases in which total removal of the lesion with its matrix was accomplished and the ossicular chain was not disrupted, follow-ups with microscopic examination should be scheduled every 6 months for the first 5 postoperative years and annually thereafter.

BACTERIAL MENINGITIS

Meningitis is primarily a disease of the CNS. More specifically, it is an inflammation of the coverings (meninges) of the brain and its circulating fluid (CSF) that may extend to adjacent organs such as the brain itself or the ear. Physicians have been aware of meningitis for centuries, but it was not until the nineteenth century that SNHL was recognized as a complication of this disease.[64]

Meningitis in the neonate may result from a maternal infection, and thus be considered congenital; however, most cases are acquired in the postnatal period. In fact, postnatal meningitis is the most common cause of acquired hearing loss in children. Since the advent of antibiotics, mortality from this disease has diminished, resulting in a statistical increase of SNHL in the survivors.

The ability of meningitis to cause neurological damage varies according to such factors as host defenses, bacterial virulence, age of the patient, time between exposure to the disease and onset of treatment, intensity of treatment, and duration of the disease.[65-69] Specifically, these criteria advert the relationship of the risk factors for hearing loss to CNS damage. An example of such a situation is the case of a child under 1 year of age whose treatment began 3 to 4 days after the onset of symptoms, and in whom the virulence of the bacteria produced a fall in the sugar content of the CSF, associated with an increase in the lactic acid content. So, while the criteria mentioned may be ideal for determination of contributing causes of hearing loss and brain damage, it is the laboratory findings of low levels of glucose and high amounts of lactic acid in the CSF that give definitive evidence of high risk for neurological damage.

Incidence

Bacterial meningitis has been the most common cause of acquired deafness in infancy and childhood. The incidence of hearing loss as a result of bacterial meningitis has not been established precisely.

Although meningitis may be viral in origin, most cases resulting in neurological deficits are caused by bacterial organisms. The bacteria involved in this disease process have generally been identified as *Haemophilus influenzae Type B (Hib)*, *Diplococcus pneumoniae*, and *Neisseria meningitidis*. These three organisms were identified, in one reported study, as the responsible agents in 89% of cases studied.[69] Of these three organisms, *Hib* has been reported to be the most common cause of meningitis (66%) and, consequently, the most common bacteria to produce hearing loss. (It must be realized that *Hib* per isolated case is not the major cause of neurologic deficit such as hearing loss, it is just that the number of cases of *Hib* have been the most common cause of meningitis. Therefore, if these are added together, they cause more hearing loss than the other organisms.) In particular, *Hib*, associated with low concentrations of CSF glucose, has been shown to be relatively more virulent and to cause more late sequelae.[65] Studies of meningococcal meningitis in children show the incidence of SNHL to be 5% in those manifesting little or no other sequelae,[70,71] which is a possible indication of this bacterial agent's susceptibility to present day antibiotics.

Of the three major bacteria currently causing meningitis, the pneumococcus is associated with the poorest prognosis with respect to both morbidity and mortality (20%).[66] Group B hemolytic streptococcus is the most frequent gram-positive organism causing meningitis in neonates.[72] Dodge states that s-pneumonia organisms in 30 patients infected showed a 31% hearing deficit, either unilateral or bilateral. N. meningitis infection occurred at 10.5% hearing deficit in 19 patients and *Hib* infection at 6% of 118 patients.[73] This study demonstrates the decrease of *Hib* meningitis resulting from the use of *H. influenzae* vaccine.

According to the Department of Health and Human Services[74] *Hib* was the leading cause of invasive bacterial disease among children in the United States. Prior to the use of effective vaccines (1990), 1 in 200 children developed invasive *Hib* by the age of 5 years. Meningitis affected 60% of these children, and 3-6% died as a result of the disease. In groups of survivors of meningitis, 20-30% developed permanent sequelae, ranging from mild hearing loss to mental retardation. Approximately two thirds of all cases of *Hib* disease affected infants and children less than 15 months of age. Prior to 1990, three *Hib* conjugate vaccines were administered to children older than 15 months of age in the United States. In 1990, there was approval of a vaccine for routine administration to infants, beginning at 2 months of age. The efficacy of these vaccines has been excellent.

Meningitis of viral origin may be the most common form of this disease; the least common form is of fungal origin.[75] It is questionable, however, that viral meningitis is a cause of acquired hearing loss in children. Although prenatal viral infections of rubella or CMV are known to cause congenital SNHL,[76] viral agents causing meningitis have not been proved to cause postnatal hearing loss. Despite accurate diagnosis, improved therapy, and a decrease in the mortality over the past decades, meningitis in children is still frequently associated with a serious compromise in hearing. Furthermore, survivors of meningitis, including some who are free of detectable hearing loss or other neurological deficits, may function at significantly lower levels of their potential than their nonmeningitic peers.[77,78] Rasmussen et al's[79] long-term study of otologic sequelae following pneumococcal meningitis studied a group of survivors 4 to 16 years following discharge from their disease. Twenty-three of these patients had otological sequelae, of which 17 were hearing losses, 9 had vertigo, and 13 had vestibular abnormalities among other symptoms referable to the nose. Among the patients with hearing loss, 4 were bilateral and 6 were unilateral deafness. Two had mild hearing loss and 5 had slight hearing loss. This study involved patients who were both children and adults.

Routes of Infections, Diagnosis, and Treatment

In the preantibiotic era, meningitis commonly arose from the invasion of the meninges by an infection of the middle ear or a brain abscess. These routes of infection are now considered rare. The most common pathway of invasion today is the bloodstream, and the most usual site of the original infection is the URI.[80] Otitis media may occur at the same time, but the two processes are independent of one another.

The symptoms of meningitis include fever, headache, neck stiffness, irritability, altered consciousness, and vomiting.[81] Microscopic examination of the CSF, achieved by a lumbar puncture (LP), is necessary to make a definitive diagnosis of meningitis. The changes in the CSF include increases in inflammatory cells (WBCs), protein, and lactic acid concentrations, and a reduction in the glucose level. The magnitude of these changes correlates generally with the severity of the disease. Extensive infiltration of the meninges and perivascular spaces by bacteria and exudate are the major pathological findings on tissue study.

Fluid for cultures of the CSF should be taken by LP. When the bacterial agent causing the infection is not known, large doses of ampicillin and chloromycetin should be given. When the results of the cultures become known, therapy with specific antibiotics may be initiated. Should the cultures show no bacterial growth, astute observation of the patient must be undertaken to determine the possible root of the infection, and cultures made of any suspected material. For example, an otitis media may be the source and, if so, immediate incision of the tympanic membrane with drainage of the tympanic cavity (tympanotomy or myringotomy) for culture is necessary.

With the presentation of symptoms of severe earache, low grade fever, headache in the area above the ear, or a pulsating pain deep in the ear, other types of otological surgery may be indicated. These procedures include a simple mastoidectomy, when there is evidence of inflammation of the mastoid cavity, or a radical mastoidectomy, when there is a keratoma or cholesteatoma (with or without an adjacent temporal bone abscess). It should be pointed out that such surgical procedures are rarely indicated today. In the case of recurrent meningitis, the presence of a labyrinthine window fistula[82-84] must be considered.

A program of prevention that has been universally applied has been inoculation with pneumococcal vaccine. However, vaccine is not available for all strains of streptococcus and, consequently, the effectiveness of this strategy is limited. The search for a vaccine effective against *Hib* has been successful. There have been disappointments in the use of the S. pneumonia vaccine in that it reduced the pneumococcal type of specific infection in vaccinated children, but has been insufficient to affect the number of episodes of infection after immunization.

Pathophysiology

It has been established that deafness resulting from meningitis is attributable to a bilateral inflammation of the membranous structures of the cochlea due to the extension of the infection from the meninges. The two recognized routes of extension are through the cochlear aqueduct[85] and along the paths of the vessels and nerves of the internal auditory canal[86,87] (Fig 5–5). Circulating bacterial toxins in the CSF enter the perilymphatic fluid system and, by absorption, enter the endolymphatic system. Temporal bone studies[88] have demonstrated significant findings. There was associated evidence of inflammation of the nerves, however, in the perineural spaces. The significance of this finding as to the cause of permanent or temporary hearing loss is unknown, especially in light of the fact that the facial nerve is undisturbed in cases of bacterial meningitis that affect these anatomical sites. Igarashi et al[89] found that the infection had invaded the striae vascularis through the bloodstream in one of five temporal bones with pneumococcal meningitis.

Subsequently, there is a replacement of the membranous labyrinth with fibrous tissue and then, in some cases, calcium is deposited and new bone is formed. Some nerve elements survive this destructive process, and this greatly enhances the potential benefits of the cochlear implant. The cause of hydrops secondary to meningitis is still to be explored.

Studies have shown that patients treated with dexamethasone at or before infusion of antibiotics tend to suffer less hearing loss. They have hypothesized that hearing loss is caused by cytokines released by the killing of bacteria by the body's defense mechanisms and antibiotics. These studies on dexamethasone originated in the late 1980s and were practiced in the early 1990s, but no further reports can be identified on the efficacy of this treatment.[90-93]

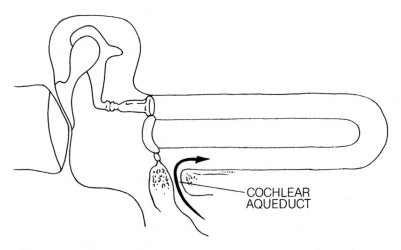

Fig 5-5.—Schematic diagram of the inner ear and cochlear aqueduct suggesting a route of bacterial invasion from the subarachnoid space to the labyrinth.

The encephalopathy (brain edema) of bacterial meningitis has been discussed in detail by Fishman and coworkers.[94] Brain edema may be defined as an increase in the brain volume secondary to an increase in its water content. When well-localized or of a mild degree, brain edema is associated with little or no clinical evidence of brain dysfunction. However, when severe it may result in major focal or generalized signs of brain dysfunction and sequelae, such as mental retardation, seizures, or hemiparesis. The animal studies of Fishman and colleagues suggest that the inflammatory exudate induces a cytotoxic edema as a result of hypoxia. The brain cells swell because of influx of tissue water brought about by the rapid accumulation of sodium within the cell structure. There is also a loss of intracellular potassium. The decrease in CSF glucose is a result of increased brain metabolism, an effect initiated by the toxin of the bacteria. The level of lactic acid, a byproduct of the increased brain metabolism, is consequently increased.

In severe cases of bacterial meningitis, the vasogenic mechanism may occur in addition to the cytotoxic mechanism. The vasogenic mechanism is characterized by increased permeability of brain capillary cells, resulting in an increase in the extracellular fluid space. This is unlike cytotoxic brain edema, in which cellular swelling and decreased extracellular fluid spaces are seen. The intake of very high dosages of the glucocorticoid dexamethasone (Decadron) has been considered of benefit in the reduction of vasogenic edema; however, there is no basis to support any beneficial effects of this therapy on cytotoxic edema.[94]

The necessary level of CSF glucose to substantiate neurological deficits is not a specific one. Statistically, a significant number of meningitic patients developed hearing impairment when their CSF glucose concentration was less than 28 mg/dl.[75]

Vestibular Involvement in Meningitis

Through history or observation, or both, infants and children with bilateral vestibular damage will show a delay in the development of gross motor skills, such as walking, standing, and sitting. They may also show positional instability, such as falling easily and stumbling. On the other hand, fine motor skills, such as in grasping and eating, may be normal. In the normal process of hearing evolvement and motor development in children, any delay in the achievement of gross motor activities commonly is interpreted as evidence of a neuromuscular disorder. Furthermore, unusually slow acquisition of motor, language, and personal-social milestones is usually interpreted as the result of "brain damage" or mental retardation. To avoid such false impressions, particularly in children who are hearing-impaired, vestibular function in infancy or childhood must be ascertained to determine the cause when such delays occur.

Vestibular testing of meningitic children should include standard ENG, especially caloric stimulation and RT. Results of the standard caloric test in children with vestibular damage show diminished activity of the labyrinth on caloric stimulation corresponding to the degree of damage. If the labyrinthine end organ has been completely destroyed by the disease, caloric activity (or response) will be absent. The response to computerized RT is measured by the degree of phase deviation to the lower frequencies on turning. In the presence of hearing loss in the post-meningitic patient, abnormal vestibular function is accurately quantified, since both labyrinths are stimulated simultaneously.[95]

Auditory Brainstem Response (ABR)

The most significant diagnostic contribution of an ABR is the verification of the presence of a central lesion, although it may not be located precisely. This procedure has been used to assess hearing loss and possible brainstem damage in patients recovering from bacterial meningitis. In the young child, ABR provides an effective method of determining hearing levels when conventional audiometric techniques are not successful.

Brainstem damage, as recorded by ABR, is most likely to be found when concomitant symptoms, such as seizures, hydrocephalus, or nerve palsies, are obvious. With these neurological signs, clear evidence of brainstem abnormalities has been reported in 10% of postmeningitic patients tested in one study.[96] In this same study, 15% of the patients tested had borderline normal ABR results. Follow-up ABR testing indicated a reversal in brainstem damage in some patients, indicating some reorganization in brainstem structures. However, ABR cannot be obtained when responses are greater than 90 dB (profound SNHL). Within these severe-to-profound thresholds, researchers have found a high number of cases of postmeningitic hearing loss, and the risk for brainstem damage in these patients could be greater.

Several ABR recordings obtained in the early stage of bacterial meningitis have revealed some important findings in a small number of patients with postmeningitic hearing impairment.[97-99] There appears to be early evidence of the hearing loss during the course of the disease, either at the time of admission to the hospital, or within the first 24 hours thereafter. There is also some indication of a crucial period during the first week of the disease that the hearing loss may either return to normal or become permanent.

Audiological Findings and Management

Hearing loss in postmeningitic children varies in amount, symmetry, and configuration of the involved frequencies (low frequency loss, flat loss, or high frequency loss). Furthermore, some patients will demonstrate a fluctuating hearing loss, and a progressive loss is common (Figs 5–6 and 5–7).

In an ongoing study of 44 ears (22 patients) at ECHO Foundation, approximately 50% (21 ears) demonstrated severe to profound SNHL secondary to meningitis. The other had mild-to-moderate SNHL. In two patients with mild moderate SNHL, hearing returned to normal a few weeks after discharge from the hospital.

Fluctuation and progression of the hearing loss occurred in 22 ears (11 patients) or 50% of the ears, including those of the two patients whose hearing had improved to normal levels. Two patients had fluctuating hearing, predominantly in the higher frequencies, that had persisted over 3 years: response to steroids (dexamethasone) has brought their hearing back to previous levels.

The fact that the hearing loss is unstable in 50% of postmeningitic children is significant. To ensure proper amplification, close monitoring of hearing levels is necessary; this should also be done in the treatment of fluctuating hearing loss. During periods of hearing fluctuation and progression, the hearing should be examined by audiometry every week; otherwise the hearing should be checked every 3 months for approximately 3 years and then, when it becomes stable, every 6 months until approximately the age of 8 years (Table 5–4).

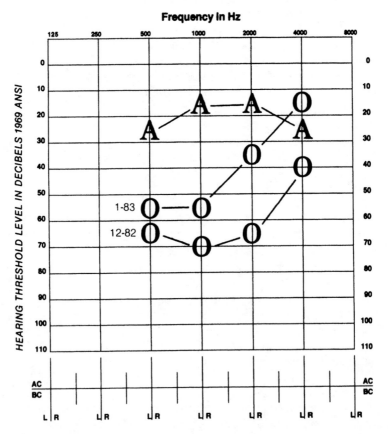

Fig 5-6.—Pure tone audiogram, right ear, showing a fluctuation of the hearing. This fluctuation occurred intermittently over a 3-year period following a meningitic infection. Thresholds of hearing have responded to treatment with cortisone. (A) represents aided binaural hearing. (O) represents unaided hearing in the right ear.

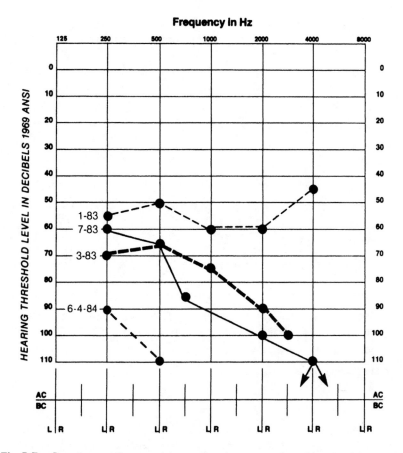

Fig 5-7.—Pure tone audiogram, right ear, showing progression of hearing loss due to meningitis.

Audiological Screening

Statistics indicate that SNHL will be a sequela in 10% of pediatric patients with bacterial meningitis. Such a significant percentage mandates that these patients be examined audiometrically prior to their discharge from the hospital. Bacterial meningitis represents a small percentage in the total of pediatric diagnoses of those children with SNHL; therefore, it is recommended that an ABR be used to evaluate these patients for SNHL. If sedation or anesthesia is undesirable because of the recent medical insult from the disease, behavioral testing by a pediatric audiologist should be employed.

Table 5–4. Audiological Recommendations for Postmeningitic Children

I. For all postmeningitic children:

1. Tympanometry before audiological evaluation to rule out conductive hearing loss.

2. Auditory brainstem response (ABR) or behavioral audiometry evaluation prior to hospital discharge.

II. For children with mild (0-35 dB) hearing loss (HL):

1. Delay amplification for 2 months.

2. Tympanograms before each audiogram.

3. Soundfield audiometry every other week for 2 months.

4. After 3 months, monthly audiological testing during first year, every 3 months during second year, then every 6 months until age 8 years; once a year thereafter.

5. Regular hearing aid checks.

III. For children with moderate (40-60 dB), severe(70-90 dB), or profound (90 dB and greater) HL:

1. Tympanograms before each pure tone or soundfield test.

2. Monthly pure tone or soundfield audiometry during first year, every 3 months during second year; then every 6 months until age 8 years; once a year thereafter.

3. Aided soundfield testing every 3 to 6 months.

4. Regular hearing aid checks.

IV. For children with asymmetrical HL regardless of degree:

1. Tympanograms before each audiogram.

2. Monthly pure tone or soundfield audiometry during first year; every 3 months during second year; then every 6 months until age 8 years; once a year thereafter.

3. Aided soundfield testing every 3 to 6 months.

4. Regular hearing aid checks.

Because hearing loss in postmeningitic children is unstable, a close monitoring system is necessary.

Screening for acoustic reflex in the postmeningitic stage has not been reported, and should be investigated. However, edema of the neurological structures in the acoustic reflex arc may preclude elicitation of accurate results.

Timing of Amplication With Hearing Aids

When a mild SNHL (0 to 35 dB) due to meningitis is identified prior to hospital discharge, amplification by hearing aids should be postponed for 2 months. Obviously, in a number of these patients, the hearing levels will return to normal, presumably as the edema of the neurological organs (eg, organ of Corti, eighth nerve) resolves. When a moderate (greater than 40 dB) to severe to profound SNHL is identified, the child should receive amplification with hearing aids immediately. There is animal laboratory evidence to substantiate the belief that atrophy of the central auditory pathway organs occurs from disuse when the peripheral organ is ablated.[100-102]

Vienny et al[97] recorded brainstem auditory evoked responses in 51 children from the initial aspect of the illness within 48 hours of establishing a diagnosis of meningitis. Evoked potential audiograms in 11 cases (21.6%) were abnormal at 48 hours, but at the time of discharge 2 weeks later, this group had recovered to normal hearing. In five cases (9.8%), the hearing impairment persisted at the time of discharge. In the remainder of the 35 cases (68.6%), the hearing was normal. These authors concluded that in this group with persistent auditory impairment, damage had occurred very early, and was irreversible from the onset. All their cases with permanent hearing deficit had suffered from H-influenza meningitis. Two were younger than 2 years of age. Kaplan et al[98] evaluated 37 children with bacterial meningitis within 48 hours of admission. Four had hearing loss detected at the time of admission. Two had hearing loss that persisted, and both losses were profound. Improvements occurred in the other two. Others have demonstrated similar findings.[103,104]

Reemphasis of Effect of Negative Pressure in SNHL

Negative middle ear pressure due to partial obstruction of the eustachian tube is found to cause low and high frequency conductive hearing loss (approximately 10 to 15 dB loss in the low frequencies and 5 dB loss in the high frequencies) in normally hearing children. Because this temporary hearing loss has little or no effect in hearing of speech sounds, it is of little consequence to the normally hearing child. However, to the hearing-impaired child, a hearing loss of 10 to 15 dB may make the difference of hearing or not hearing speech (Table 5-5).

Other Meningitic Disabilities

Meningitic hearing loss may be found in conjunction with other disabilities. When the inflammatory process of meningitis affects the brain and meninges, it is referred to as meningoencephalitis. The sequelae resulting from this insult to the brain can be identified by neurological and EEG studies. The symptoms of such damage include seizure disorders, emotional problems, paresis, and visual impairment.

Table 5–5. Recommendation Based on Tympanometry and SNHL

1. Negative pressure greater than –50 mm of water (mm H$_2$O): refer to otologist for medical treatment

2. Negative pressure of greater than –50 mm H$_2$O for more than 4 weeks despite medication: refer to otologist for myringotomy with tubes.

3. If the child has greater than –50 mm H$_2$O at the time of audiological testing, reschedule audiological evaluation for 1 week later, after the child has been on medication for the week.

4. If the child has tubes at the time of audiological testing, test on impedance bridge to see if tubes are patent. If one or both tubes do not open, refer to otologist for treatment. Reschedule audiological testing for 1 week later.

There are other postmeningitic disabilities that, although not subclinical signs, cannot be elicited by routine testing procedures. Yet the educational and psychological impact of these disabilities dramatically affect the learning progress of a child. In the 22 children who were postmeningitic studied at ECHO, such disabilities included (in addition to a hearing impairment) motor problems, hyperactivity, and auditory processing problems. These psychoneurological-social defects result in probable reduced intellectual functioning (Table 5–6).

Motor Problems

Vestibular damage reflected in deviant motor behavior has been alluded to earlier. Realistically, deviant motor behavior in children would be regarded as a disability only when it grossly imposes on their motor capacities. One child of the 22 in the ECHO sample exhibited such a motor symptom, whereas in the others, symptoms were typically vestibular in origin, and these children showed difficulty with equilibrium in various ways. Generalized clumsiness and specific motor skills, such as walking and sitting up, will often need to be corrected or redeveloped when these children enter a rehabilitation program. Other "soft" signs of motor inabilities may not be vestibular in origin. These include poor coordination of finer movements, such as are required in building with blocks, inability to form or recall motor patterns (apraxia), and inability to focus the eyes for an extended period of time. In this regard, additional soft signs, such as left-right confusion and overall slow maturation, may be similar to those of developmental lags. For children who show such difficulties, sensorimotor integration (occupational therapy) may be helpful.

Table 5–6. Most Common Factors that Affect Learning in the Postmeningitic Hearing-Impaired Child

1. Hearing loss.

2. Motor problems, gross or fine; overall awkwardness or loss of coordination.

3. Hyperactive behavior: stress, anxiety, poor attention span.

4. Visual problems.

5. Auditory processing problems: inconsistent responses to sound that should be audible based on aided hearing; inability to learn meaning of sounds.

6. Seizure disorders: may be subtle, as localized tremors, blank looks, or staring.

7. Emotional problems: inappropriate laughter, sobbing, and so forth.

8. Retardation.

9. Paresis.

Hyperactivity

Many children with hearing impairment have a tendency to be hyperactive, probably because diminished auditory input causes inattention followed by compensation, resulting in overreaction in behavior. Hyperactivity, short attention span, stress, and anxiety prevalent in children with postmeningitic SNHL are helped by occupational therapy or medication. During therapy sessions, activities should be varied and directed toward increasing the attention span of the child. For obvious reasons, surrounding distractions should be held to a minimum during therapy sessions.

Auditory Processing Disorders

Observation of children with postmeningitic SNHL has revealed that many of them have auditory learning disorders, probably due to CNS deficits. Such children may not associate words they have been deemed able to hear (on the basis of aided audiograms) with the appropriate meanings of the words. Although these children may be able to detect and hear speech or environmental sounds, they appear to have poor memory or recall, inability to associate the word learned with the experience, and inconsistencies in response to sound (ie, responding correctly to a sound one moment, only to not respond to the same sound moments later).

The children in the ECHO sample have not been tested for minimal neurological deficits that might cause disabilities in reading, writing, spelling, and arithmetic because of the age and stage of development.

Impaired Intellectual Function

As a rule, nonverbal tests must be used to evaluate the intellectual functioning of children with postmeningitic SNHL. Therefore, the similarities and differences between verbal and nonverbal tests must be evaluated critically. Inasmuch as the results of these tests correlate significantly, it is apparent that they measure different aspects of intelligence.[105] Among the 22 ECHO children, 4 have been tested with the nonverbal Kaufmann Assessment Battery and the Leiter International Performance Scale. For comparative reasons, 4 children with nonmeningitic hearing impairment children in the same age group were also tested. The results for these two small groups were essentially the same; the average score for the children with postmeningitic hearing impairment was 107 and the average score for the children with nonmeningitic hearing impairment was 104. No conclusions could be drawn from this small group of children, but it is believed that if a child is not making adequate progress, regardless of the teaching method employed, nonverbal psychological testing should be undertaken.

Recommendations

Not all patients with postmeningitic SNHL have learning disabilities. Some make adequate progress and perform well. Because most of these patients have acquired deafness and have experienced normal hearing, it is generally agreed that beneficial teaching should start with auditory training; that is, the development of residual hearing and listening skills. Evaluation of the child's progress and of the potential for ultimate success should be made every 6 months to determine if auditory teaching is to be continued. If the decision is that the auditory modality is not to be continued, it is recommended that at the 12- or 18-month evaluation stage, the auditory-oral method be used, followed by cued speech and then signing.

Monitoring of hearing levels has been outlined earlier in this book. Every effort should be made to identify any changes in the hearing levels as well as any psychoneurological or psychosocial disabilities secondary to meningitis (Fig 5–7).

In terms of the psychology of hearing impairment, the hearing loss due to meningitis presents many avenues for repercussion. The diverse effects of this disease on the auditory organ and CNS make each person's situation unique, and careful diagnosis is crucial in the development of an effective education program. The clinician must investigate beyond the peripheral hearing loss for any behavior indicative of other sequelae of the disease (Fig 5–8).

PERILYMPH FISTULA IN CHILDREN
WITH PREEXISTING SNHL

Investigation of CSF otorrhea has been a major interest in modern otology. CSF may reach the middle ear either directly through a defect in the tegmen of the bone (typically, this is more common in adults), or when a perilymph fistula (PLF) is present via the labyrinth. The most frequent middle ear leakage sites are the stapes footplate or annular ligament (Fig 5–9).

In the past, a child with recurrent meningitis, typically pneumococcal, and a unilateral or bilateral deafness, was the clinical setting for an endaural CSF fistula. Typically, the meningitis would have been recurrent and the first bout could have been as early as age 1 month. In such a case, labyrinthine malformations would have been common and of course, accompanied by SNHL in infants and children, has been considered by some an indication for a tympanotomy to rule out the presence of a peri-

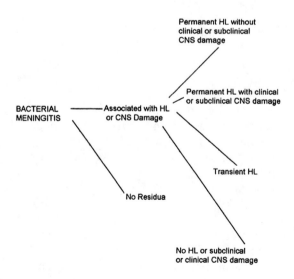

Fig 5-8.—Postmeningitic flow pattern.

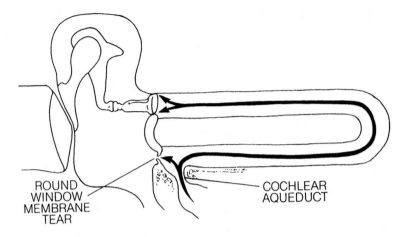

ROUND
WINDOW
MEMBRANE
TEAR

COCHLEAR
AQUEDUCT

Fig 5-9.—Schematic diagram of middle and inner ear showing possible pathogenesis of injury to round and oval window membranes as a result of sudden increases in fluid pressures through the cochlear aqueduct.

lymphatic fistula. In 1988 we reported[106] on the exploration of 36 ears in 26 children with progressive-type SNHL and found a perilymphatic fistula in 4 ears (11%). Although there was radiographic evidence of inner ear deformity in one half of these children, a definite fistula was found in only 4 of 18 radiographically abnormal ears explored (22%). Even in the 4 patients with a history of a "traumatic event" that could implicate a fistula such as exertional barotrauma, a fistula was found in only 1. One should accept the fact, therefore, that there are a number of possible causes for progression of preexisting SNHL, and surgical exploration of the middle ear is not recommended on the basis of progression alone. Instead, exploration of the suspected PLF should be strongly considered when there is the history of an "event," and/or radiographic evidence of inner ear abnormalities. As a result of this study, we started to recommend that any patient with congenital inner ear defects avoid potential fistula-producing activities, such as contact sports, weight lifting, kayaking, scuba diving, sky diving, and deep diving into a pool. We also caution against vigorous nose blowing, coughing, sneezing, and straining with constipation when possible. The likelihood of a fistula developing in a pediatric patient with a SNHL, but no congenital inner ear abnormality, is no greater than any child in the normal population; therefore, such precautions are not necessary.

One must advise the parents that even when a fistula is present and repair has been accomplished, that it has been shown that only a mild effect on hearing improvement may be present. More importantly, it should be stressed that repair of such a fistula would tend to prevent progression of the hearing loss. Typically, vertigo, when present, is totally relieved.

The difficulty is in deciding which patients have a fistula caused by pressure breaks and which do not. In at least one-third of adults the condition was of "spontaneous" onset; therefore, historical evidence of trauma or stress is not always present. Nevertheless, all patients with activity-related SNHL, a history of disequilibrium with SNHL,[107] or progressive hearing loss superimposed on a preexisting SNHL, may be suspected of having a perilymph fistula.

Assessment

Audiometric variance is common in infants and children with a perilymph fistula. There is no typical configuration to the hearing loss; that is, fluctuating, progressive, sudden onset, and nonchanging hearing losses, as well as normal hearing, may be found.[108]

Vestibular function tests, using the fistula test with Frenzel glasses and negative pressure (Fig 5–10), has been of value in identifying these fistulae in adults.[109] The value of this test procedure in children having fistulae is yet to be demonstrated. A positive Hennebert sign (Fig 5–10) or symptoms elicited by a fistula test with Frenzel glasses will not be identified by ENG, as the identifying sign is an eye movement or deviation, not a nystagmus.

SNHL and recurring meningitis are more prevalent among patients with middle or inner ear defects.[110-112] Patients with a Mondini defect, occurring in syndromes or in isolation, have been shown to have histological anomalies of the footplate of the stapes.[113] Although radiography may demonstrate normal bony structures, less conspicuous deformities cannot be identified. Abnormalities of the labyrinthine windows have often been encountered on exploratory tympanotomy, including one that was an incomplete niche of the round window facing laterally rather than posteriorly.[114] Confirmation of a sudden hearing loss, a slow progressive hearing loss, or radiographic findings of inner ear defects, are the most presumptive signs of a perilymphatic fistula in young children. The predisposition of young children to spasms of coughing and of older children to head injury and stress activity adds to the clinical picture.

In summary, congenital perilyphatic fistula is more likely to be associated with temporal bone or extracranial abnormalities, such as a Mondini malformation, or any condition that is associated with middle ear abnormalities.[115]

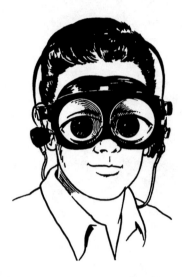

Fig 5-10.—Fistula test with Frenzel glasses and a tympanometer. This test is done in darkness. Tympanometer pressure is increased to plus 500 mm H_2O, then decreased to minus 500 mm H_2O. An eye deviation, elicited by negative pressure, is indicative of a positive fistula test (positive Hennebert sign). A sensation or dizziness or nausea, in the absence of eye deviation, indicates a positive Hennebert's symptom.

Prevention

Patients with inner ear defects or proven perilymphatic fistulae would appear to be at high risk for sudden or progressive hearing loss and should, therefore, be restricted from activities that would place stress on their inner ears. Such activities would include weight lifting, strenuous calisthenics, scuba and deep water diving, parachuting, skiing, boxing, wrestling, karate, and flying in nonpressurized aircraft. Also to be avoided are hobbies or occupations involving environmental pressurization, firearms, the use of compressors, and so forth. URIs should be treated promptly to avoid development of coughs and ear infections. Such implements as cotton-tipped applicators should be avoided by the patient because of the possibility of causing direct trauma.

Surgical Management

To prevent pooling of the local anesthetic in the labyrinthine window areas, the vascular area is not injected. Tympanotomy incisions are extended to the anterior canal landmarks and a wide tympanotomy flap is elevated to expose the tympanum as much as possible. It is imperative that the middle ear remain dry; even a tiny amount of blood or local anesthetic will obscure a minute perilymph fistula.

While visualizing the labyrinthine windows, the clinician should make an attempt to provoke leakage from the fistula site with a Valsalva test and coughing. To accomplish this in children under general anesthesia, the anesthesia should be lightened and coughing provoked.

There are two membranes within the niche of the round window (Fig 5–11). One is the membrane of the niche and the other is the membrane of the window, which is the true membrane. Do not mistake the niche membrane for the true membrane. The niche membrane may be reticulated, have a single perforation, have a network of many perforations, or be a closed type, without any perforation. The true membrane is located deep in the round window niche. It is mobile and, if ruptured, will have a slit rather than a perforation.[116] At times the bony niche overhang must be removed with a small curette to visualize the true round window membrane. The incudostapedial joint should be pumped gently while the round window membrane and the stapedial footplate are visualized. Fistulae of the round window are uncommon. Exposure to the posterior footplate may require removal of the bony external canal edge superior to the chorda tympani nerve. An attempt should be made to visualize all areas of the footplate while gently pumping the incudostapedial joint. If a fistula is found, the mucous membrane of the surrounding bony area should be elevated gently. Perichondrium from the tragus is usually adequate to cover fistulae and the area beyond. Large size pieces of Gelfoam should be packed around the graft and stacked to the eardrum to prevent it from slipping out of place.

In addition to the oval and round windows, the area of the fissula ante fenestram should also be observed. Patency may persist as late as the second year of childhood or even into adulthood.[117] A thickening, or localized edema, overlying the fissula ante fenestram may be a sign of perilymphatic leakage. The area posterior and superior to the round window should be observed for a fissure or bony cleft. If no fistula is found, but the historical and physical evidence is extenuating, a graft should be applied to the superior and inferior aspects of the footplate and the area of the fissula ante fenestram.

Microfissures in human temporal bones have been found superior and inferior to the oval window; however, the histogenesis of these defects is unknown.[118] Studies in guinea pigs in which a single electrode cochlear microphonic recording was used have shown only slight SNHL when the round window membrane was ruptured.[119] The evidence presented in this study indicates that there is underlying pathology in the membranous cochlea in cases of more severe hearing loss.

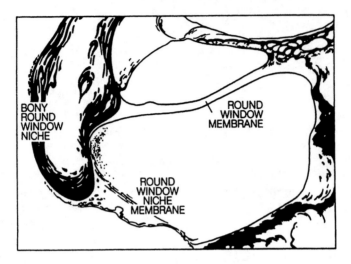

Fig 5-11.—The round window membrane and the round window niche membrane. To observe the round window membrane a small portion of the niche of the round window may need to be removed with a stapes curette. (Drawn from Y. Nomura.[116] Reprinted with permission.)

Results

In adults, hearing improvement following fistula closure is statistically less than 50%,[121] vestibular symptoms are abated, and recurrence rate may be high (30%), according to R. Kohut (personal communication).

Progression of SNHL in infants and children experiencing activity-related hearing loss or inner ear defects is an indication for emergency tympanotomy. However, this author saw no impressive evidence of improved hearing in such patients in a group of 18 young children with congenital SNHL. A definite fistula was found in only two ears in this group; one in a patient who had coughing spasms followed by increased hearing thresholds, and the other in a patient with a Mondini syndrome. The variance in preoperative audiograms and audiograms obtained post-operatively at 3 months, 6 months, and 12 months for the frequencies of 250 to 4000 Hz, was analyzed statistically. Using a 5% level of significance, no differences were indicated in the hearing thresholds at any frequency. Stabilization of hearing has been noted at 1 year postoperatively, but more time is needed to verify this (author's statistics).

AUTOIMMUNE INNER EAR DISEASE

Recent observations have led to the conclusion that immunological activity in the ear is often overlooked as the cause of a disease process. Localized examples of immunological ear disease, some hypothetical, include tympanosclerosis, autoimmune inner ear disease, middle ear effusion, and granular myringitis,[121,122] a rejection reaction seen in some cases of tympanoplasty. In some patients, there is evidence that ear symptoms are likely to be a part of a systemic immune complex disorder, such as rheumatoid arthritis, lupus erythematosus, or some other autoimmune disease. In 1979, autoimmune inner ear disease was proposed by McCabe[123] as a diagnostic entity on the clinical basis that, in 18 patients, a dramatic improvement of hearing was obtained with treatment.

A cruel mistake is the end result of autoimmune disease. The patient's immune defenders, especially the T-cells, attack the very tissues they should protect. In inner ear disease, it is the labyrinth. In rheumatoid arthritis, it is the joints. In diabetes it is the pancreas, and in multiple sclerosis, it is the brain and spinal cord. Why these T-cells become traitors is unknown.

Clinical Picture

A SNHL of autoimmune origin is characterized by rapid onset with progression, often with significant fluctuations, over a period of weeks to months. This pattern can usually be distinguished from that of a SNHL attributable to other causes:

1. Head injuries and blast injuries result in SNHL of immediate onset that progresses rapidly over a period of hours to days.
2. Ototoxicity and labyrithine inflammation both produce SNHL of rapid onset that also progresses over a period of hours or days.
3. Presbycusis and noise-induced SNHL have a gradual onset and progress slowly (over a period of years).
4. Otosclerosis typically produces a conductive hearing loss, but may cause SNHL that develops and slowly progresses over a period of years.

The hearing loss seen in autoimmune SNHL most commonly mimics that seen in Ménière's disease, except that it is slightly more exaggerated and more rapidly progressive.

Most cases of autoimmune inner ear disease reported so far have been in adults. When this disease is suspected in children, delayed hereditary SNHL and luetic labyrinthitis must be excluded as diagnoses. In those conditions, the hearing loss is much more gradual than in autoimmune SNHL, occurring over a period of months to years. Autoimmune SNHL appears to follow the same statistical distribution as autoimmune diseases in general. Middle-aged women are by far the most vulnerable, with an average age of 44 years (range of 6-76 years) at initial evaluation.[124] SNHL has been reported to occur in association with, or secondary to, a variety of other autoimmune diseases, such as those outlined in Table 5–7. Systemic immunologic disorders that produce otologic disorders have been reviewed by others.[132] Hughes et al[124] reported that 25% to 30% of their patients had systemic immune disease. We have not found nearly that large a percentage, but continue to test for concomitant systemic immune disorders.

Effusion of the middle ear may precede or accompany the SNHL, which is progressive, and may drop rather precipitously over a period of weeks or months. Variations in audiometric configuration (such as fluctuation, asymmetry, and sudden unilateral hearing loss) are common. Discrimination scores tend to remain in alignment with the amount of pure tone hearing thresholds. Progression of the hearing loss to thresholds exceeding those discernible by audiometry may also be part of this clinical picture. Although this progressive, or fluctuating, hearing loss will not respond to conventional therapy, the symptoms tend to improve with steroid therapy in cases of autoimmune inner ear disease.

Patients with autoimmune inner ear disease have peripheral vestibular lesions and reduced or absent activity on caloric vestibular testing. Rotation tests demonstrate the degree of remaining function, which can be quantified as follows: abnormal phase (leads) and absence of asymmetry (preponderance).

So far, most of the reported cases of autoimmune inner ear disease have involved adults. When the condition is suspected in children, delayed congenital SNHL and luetic labyrinthitis must be excluded as the diagnosis. A hearing loss associated with immune inner ear disease occurs over a period of weeks to months; when associated with luetic labyrinthitis or representing a delayed congenital SNHL, it may occur over a period of months to years. Obviously, a positive FTA-ABS test result will confirm presence of luetic labyrinthitis.

Laboratory Tests

There is no definite serologic test that diagnoses autoimmune inner ear disease, and most patients suspected of having this condition undergo

Table 5–7. Examples of Diseases That May Produce Primary or Secondary Autoimmune-like Sensorineural Hearing Loss [128]

Disease	Primary Targets	Ear Manifestations	Possible Diagnostic Antigens and Marker Assays
Rheumatoid arthritis (RA)	Connective tissue	CHL (involvement of the incudomalleal and incudostapedial articulations) [126]	Collagens I-IV; IgG rheumatoid factor; SS-DNA; cytoskeletal proteins
Still's disease	Connective tisssue	Same as above rheumatoid factor; autoreactive T cells	Collagens I & II; IgM
Multiple sclerosis	White matter of the brain, spinal cord	May affect balance and hearing	Myelin basic protein
Wegener's granulomatosis	Vasculitis of the upper and lower airway; kidneys	OME (encroachment on eustachian tube); SNHL(otitis media or invasive granuloma)	Neutrophil cytoplasm
Polyarteritis nodosa	Widespread necrotizing vasculitis	OME, mixed [127]; predominantly CHL [128]	Unknown
Cogan's syndrome	Interstitial keratitis	SNHL (unilateral and bilateral); tinnitus; severe vertigo [129]	Unknown (possible collagen II)
Vogt-Koyanagi-Herada syndrome	Uveitis	SNHL	Unknown

continued

Table 5–7. Continued

Disease	Primary Targets	Ear Manifestations	Possible Diagnostic Antigens and Marker Assays
Relapsing polychondritis	Multiple cartilages	Hyperemic and edematous auricles; hearing loss (pure conductive, pure sensorineural, or mixed)[130]	Collagen II
Hashimoto's thyroiditis	Thyroid	Myxedema giving the impression of hearing loss	Thyroid cell growth promoting (TSI) antibody (antigen unknown); thyrotropin receptor possible
Systemic lupus erythematosis	Virtually any tissue	CHL and SNHL[131] DNA, ribonucleoteins	Subcellular organelles,
Psoriasis	Skin	Dry rash affecting ear canal skin	Possible overprodution of transforming growth factor -B
Alport's	Basement membrane (kidney)	SNHL	Collagen IV; no antibody

Note: CHL, conductive hearing loss; OME, otitis media with effusion, SNHL, sensorineural hearing loss. From English (I)39:1-10, 1995. Used with permission.

only conventional laboratory evaluation for known autoantibodies. The usual tests include assays for erythrocyte sedimentation rate, complete blood count, cryoglobulins, circulating immune complexes, complement levels, serum protein electrophoresis, antinuclear antibody, antineutrophil cytoplasmic antibody, and rheumatoid factor. Some laboratories (eg, Inova Diagnostics and Specialty Labs) are currently attempting to develop tests to subcategorize autoantibodies based on cellular and extracellular immunofluorescent staining. These tests will, at times, give supportive evidence of a general autoimmune condition. From time to time these patients are subjected to more elaborate and specific laboratory tests, which must be regarded as research, in the hope that one or another will yield useful information. Such tests include detection of serum autoantibodies to collagen and to solubilized cochlear extracts and analysis of the T–lymphocyte transformation response to these antigens. Only highly specialized laboratories typically perform such tests.

Until more definitive criteria are established, diagnosis of autoimmune inner ear disease is based on the patient's history and response to treatment. Because of the similarities of autoimmune inner ear disease and Ménière's disease, patients with exaggerated Ménière's disease should be suspected of having autoimmune inner ear disease. If a diagnosis of progressive bilateral SNHL is not clearcut, it is advisable to institute a trial treatment for autoimmune inner ear disease, before all hearing is lost.[133]

Treatment

There are three major alternatives for treatment available for patients with autoimmune inner ear disease: (1) steroids, (2) cytotoxic drugs, and (3) plasmapheresis.

Most patients respond to short-term, high doses of dexamethasone, followed by maintenance dosages over a period of months; however, some do not, despite the amount of cortisone involved. When the cortisone is effective, the drug reduces the vasogenic edema[94] caused by the vasculitis associated with the immune complex-mediated labyrinthine tissue. Unfortunately, the complications of steroid therapy may be troublesome, especially in children. Nevertheless, hearing gain can be dramatic within days or weeks following steroid therapy.

Treatment must be altered according to failure of response with steroid or cytotoxic drugs while keeping in mind that hearing gain may not be realized until after months of continuous steroid therapy. If a patient's symptoms worsen during steroid therapy, or if toxicity and other side effects are intolerable, the use of cytotoxic drugs may be another option. The use of cytotoxic drugs is more justified in patients who are beyond reproductive age (approximately 45 years), if these agents are not contraindicated by other factors. Because they have the potential to affect reproductive cells, their use in younger patients is not recommended. However, these drugs provide effective treatment of some autoimmune inner ear diseases because of their ability to rapidly destroy activated lymphocytes to mitosis. Because of the intricate nature of such chemotherapy, consultation with a hematologist-oncologist is advised before initiation of treatment.

When steroids have been ineffective in patients who are of reproductive age, apheresis can provide yet another treatment option. Two apheresis procedures can be used[125]: (1) simple plasmapheresis, in which only plasma proteins (including autoantibodies and immune complexes) are removed and exchanged for an isotonic albumin solution; and (2) lymphoplasmapheresis, in which mononuclear cells (including autoreactive T and B lymphocytes) are also removed. The effects of apheresis are, in general, only temporary. However, the benefits are occasionally longer lasting and, in some of these cases, the use of steroids may further prolong the effects. The typical lymphoplasmapheresis regimen is to remove one to one and one half of the plasma volume every other day for five to six treatments (for example, three times a week for 2 weeks). An attempt is made to remove and exchange the entire plasma pool. The number of lymphocytes removed varies from patient to patient.

More often than not, lymphoplasmapheresis produces good results in a short period of time. The greatest deterrent to its use today is third-party payers—that is, those insurance companies that defer cooperation in providing this treatment until bureaucratic requirements can be met. By the time these requirements have been fulfilled (a matter of weeks to months), the hearing loss will have become too severe to alleviate.

When treating autoimmune inner ear disease, it must be remembered that it is a tissue-destroying condition. Early diagnosis and early intervention are essential to effective therapy. Unless the hearing loss is total, aggressive therapy can arrest or improve audiovestibular function. The therapeutic modality selected must be designed for the individual patient, promptly introduced, and thoroughly carried out under close surveillance and monitoring.

SNHL in Children With Autoimmune Inner Ear Disease

What part does autoimmune inner ear disease play in acquired hearing impairment or progressive hearing loss in childhood? At this time, there is no evidence that directly indicts this disease process as a cause of SNHL in children. The evidence supporting the hypothesis of such a cause and effect is purely clinical and is implied only by the response of 28 children to treatment with corticosteroids. Steroids were used in many children of various ages who had preexisting mild to moderate or severe hearing loss that progressed. In many instances, the hearing improved, but in most not quite to previous threshold levels. Is this a form of autoimmune inner ear disease? Probably not; there may be some infectious immune response to treatment.

Autoimmune SNHL is relatively rare, but it can be devastating in children. Early recognition and proper treatment may prevent chronic disability from a delay in speech and language development as a result of such a hearing loss.

REFERENCES

1. Downs MP, Jafek B, Wood RP. Comprehensive treatment of children with recurrent serous otitis media. *Otolaryngol Head Neck Surg.* 1981;89:658-665.
2. Freeman BA, Parkins C. The prevalence of middle ear disease among learning impaired children. *Clin Pediatr.* 1979;18:205-212.
3. Goycoolea MV, Meyerhoff WL. Otitis media. In: Meyerhoff WL, ed. *Diagnosis and Management of Hearing Loss.* Philadelphia, Pa: WB Saunders; 1984; 1143-1164.
4. Weit RJ, DeBlanc GB, Stewart J, Weider DJ. Natural history of otitis media in the American native. In: Recent Advances in Otitis Media with Effusion. *Ann Otol Rhinoi Laryngol.* 1980;89(suppl 68):1419.
5. Downs MP. Identification of children at risk for middle ear effusion problems. *Ann Otol Rhinol Laryngol.* 1980;89(suppl 68):168-171.
6. Paradise JL. Inadequate resolution of acute otitis media following antimicrobial therapy. *Pediatr Ann.* 1984;13:382-390.
7. Balkany TJ, Downs MP, Jafek BW, Krajacek MJ. Otologic manifestations in Down's syndrome. *Surg Forum.* 1978;29:582-585.
8. Balkany TJ, Downs MP, Jafek BW, Krajacek MJ. Hearing loss in Down's syndrome. *Clin Pediatr.* 1979;18:116-118.
9. Swartz DM, Swartz RH. Acoustic impedance and otoscopic findings in young children with Down's syndrome. *Arch Otolaryngol.* 1978;104:652-656.
10. Telle, DW, Klein JO, Rosner BA. Epidemiology of otitis media in children. *Ann Rhinol Laryngol.* 1980;89(suppl 68):5-6.
11. Menyuk P. Effect of persistent otitis media on language development. *Ann Otol Rhinol Laryngol.* 1980;89(suppl 69):257-263.
12. Howie VM, Ploussard JH, Sloyer J. The "otitis-prone" condition. *Am J Dis Child.* 1975;129:676-678.
13. Meyerhoff WL, Kim D, Paparella M. Pathology of chronic otitis media. *Ann Otol Rhinol Laryngol.* 1978;87:749-760.

14. Paparella M, Goycoolea MV, Meyerhoff W. Inner ear pathology and otitis media: a review. *Ann Otol Rhinol Laryngol.* 1980;89(suppl 68):249-253.
15. Paparella M, Goycoolea M, Shea D, Meyerhoff W. Endolymphatic hydrops in otitis media. *Laryngoscope.* 1979;89:43-54.
16. Brookhouser P, Worthington D, Kelly W. Middle ear disease in young children with sensorineural hearing loss. *Laryngoscope.* 1993;103:371-378.
17. Pappas Ear Clinic unpublished data.
18. Cooper JC, Langley LR, Meyerhoff WL, Gates GA. The significance of negative middle ear pressure. *Laryngoscope.* 1976;87:92-97.
19. Ling D, Ling AH. Aural Habilitation: *The Foundations of Verbal Learning in Hearing-Impaired Children.* Washington, DC: Alexander Graham Bell Association for the Deaf; 1978.
20. Klein, JO. Microbiology of otitis media. *Ann Otol Rhinol Laryngol.* 1980;89 (suppl 68):98-101.
21. Balkany TJ, Berman SA, Simmons MA, Jafek BW. Middle ear effusions in neonates. *Laryngoscope.* 1978;88:398-405.
22. Teele DW, Healy GB, Tally FP. Persistent effusions of the middle ear: cultures for anaerobic bacteria. *Ann Otol Rhinol Laryngol.* 1980;89(suppl 68):102-103.
23. Grundfast KM. A review of the efficacy of systemically administered decongestant in the prevention and treatment of otitis media. *Otolaryngol Head Neck Surg.* 1981;89:432-439.
24. Henderson FW, Collier AM, Sanyal JA, et al. A longitudinal study of respiratory viruses and bacteria in the etiology of acute otitis media with effusion. *N Engl J Med.* 1982;306:1377-1383.
25. Klein JO. Antimicrobial prophylaxis for recurrent acute otitis media. *Pediatr Ann.* 1984;13:398-403.
26. Shurin PA, Manchant CD, Kim CH. Emergence of beta-lactamase-producing strains of Branhamella catorrhalis as important agents of acute otitis media. *Pediatr Infect Dis.* 1983;2:34-38.
27. Schwartz RH. Bacteriology of otitis media: a review. *Otolaryngol Head Neck Surg.* 1981;89:444-450.
28. Holmquist J, Renvall U, Svendson P. Eustachian tube function and retraction of the tympanic membrane. *Ann Otol Rhinol Laryngol.* 1980;89(suppl 68): 65-66.
29. Beery QC, Doyle WJ, Bluestone CD, et al. Eustachian tube function in an American Indian population. *Ann Otol Rhinol Laryngol.* 1980;89(suppl 68): 28-33.
30. Bylander A, Tjernstrom O, Ingvarsson A, Ingvarsson L. Eustachian tube function in children with and without otologic history. In: Lim DJ, Bluestone CD, Klein JO, Nelson J, eds. *Proceedings of the Third International Symposium: Recent Advances in Otitis Media with Effusion.* Philadelphia, Pa: BC Decker; 1983;56-58.
31. Suzuki M, Kawauchi H, Ueyama S, et al. Immune mediated otitis media with effusion. In: Lim DJ, ed. *Recent Advances in Otitis Media,* Philadelphia, Pa: BC Decker; 1988;191-196.

32. Mogi G. Immunologic and allergic aspects of otitis media. In: Lim DJ, ed. *Recent Advances in Otitis Media*. Philadelphia, Pa: BC Decker; 1993;145-151.

33. Pelton SI, Teele DW, Reimer CB, et al. Immunologic characteristics of children with frequent recurrence of otitis media. In: Lim DJ, ed. *Recent Advances in Otitis Media*. Philadelphia, Pa: BC Decker; 1988;143-146.

34. Stenfors LE, Räusänen S. Is attachment of bacteria to the epithelial cells of the nasopharynx the key to otitis media? *Int J Pediat Otorhinol*. 1991;22:1-8.

35. Stenfors LE, Räusänen S. Occurrence of Streptococcus pneumoniae and Haemophilus influenzae in otitis media with effusion. *Clin Otol*. 1992;17: 195-199.

36. Oversen T, Ledet T. Bacteria and endotoxin in middle ear fluid and the course of secretory otitis media. *Clin Otol*. 1992;17:531-534.

37. DeMaria TF, Briggs BR, Lim DJ. Experimental otitis media with effusion following middle ear inoculation of nonviable H. influenzae. *Ann Otol Rhinol Laryngol*. 1984;93:52-56.

38. Okazaki N, DeMaria TF, Briggs BR, Lim DJ. Experimental otitis media with effusion induced by nonviable Haemophilus influenzae: cytologic study. *Am J Otol*. 1984;5:80-92.

39. Roydhouse N. Adenoidectomy for otitis media with mucoid effusion. *Ann Otol Rhinol Laryngol*. 1980;89(suppl 68):312-315.

40. Marshak G, Neriah ZB. Adenoidectomy versus tympanostomy in chronic secretory otitis media. *Ann Otol Rhinol Laryngol*. 1980;89(suppl 68):316-318.

41. Gates G, Avery CA, Prihoda TJ, Cooper JC. Effectiveness of adenoidectomy and tympanostomy tubes in the treatment of chronic otitis media with effusion. *New Eng J of Med*. 1987;317:1444-1451.

42. Browning CG, Gatehouse SG. A randomized study of the surgical management of children with persistent otitis media with effusion associated with a hearing impairment. *Journal of Laryngology and Otology*. 1993;187:284-189.

43. Pillsbury HC, Kveton JF, Saski CT, Frazier W. Quantitative bacteriology in adenoid tissue. *Otolaryngol Head Neck Surg*. 1981;89:355-363.

44. Cantekin EL, Rockette HE, Bluestone CD, Beery QC. Effect of decongestant v. with or without antihistamine on eustachian tube function. *Ann Otol Rhinol Laryngol*. 1980;89(suppl 68):290-295.

45. Bluestone CD. State of the art: definitions and classifications. In: Lim DJ, Bluestone CD, Klein JP, Nelson J, eds. *Proceedings of the Third International Symposium; Recent Advances in Otitis Media with Effusion*. Philadelphia, Pa: BC Decker; 1983;2.

46. Caparosa RJ. Comment. *Ann Otol*. 1981;90:6.

47. Mandel EM, Bluestone CD, Paradise JL, et al. Efficacy of myringotomy with and without tympanotomy tube insertion in the treatment of chronic otitis media with effusion in infants and children: results for the first year of a randomized clinical trial. In: Lim DJ, Bluestone CD, Klein JO, Nelson J, eds. *Proceedings of the Third International Symposium: Recent Advances in Otitis Media with Effusion*. Philadelphia, Pa: BC Decker; 1983:308-312.

48. Pappas DG. Triflanged tube for chronic serous otitis media. *Ann Otol Rhinol Laryngol.* 1976;82:100-101.
49. Meyerhoff WL, Giebink GS, Shea DA, Le CT. Effect of tympanostomy tubes in the pathogenesis of acute otitis media. *Am J Otolaryngol.* 1982;3:189-195.
50. Kokko E, Palva T. Clinical results and complications of tympanotomy. *Ann Otol Rhinol Laryngol.* 1976;85(suppl 25):277-279.
51. Herzon FS. Tympanotomy tubes: infectious complications. *Arch Otolaryngol* 1980;106:645-647.
52. Armstrong W, Armstrong RB. Chronic nonsuppurative otitis media. *Ann Otol Rhinol Laryngol.* 1981;90:553-535.
53. Schwartz RH, Rodriguez WJ. Draining ears in acute otitis media. Reliability of cultures. *Laryngoscope.* 1980;90:1717-1719.
54. Andersen RG, Wright CG, Meyerhoff WL. Inflammatory effects of otic drops on the middle ear. In: Lim DJ, Bluestone CD, Klein JO, Nelson J, eds. *Proceedings of the Third International Symposium: Recent Advances in Otitis Media with Effusion.* Philadelphia, Pa: BC Decker; 1983:312-315.
55. Lundy L, Graham M. Ototoxicity and ototopical medications: a survey of otolaryngologists. *Amer J of Otology.* March 1993;14(No 2):141-146.
56. Linda TE, Wicky ZS, Brandle P. Ototoxicity of eardrops, a clinical perspective. *Am J of Otol.* 1995;16(No 5):653-657.
57. Ikeda K, Morizono T, Juhn S. Cochleotoxicity of otic drops in the chinchilla: comparative study of Bestron and Cortisporin. *Am J of Otol.* 1991;12(No 6): 429-434.
58. House JW, Sheehy JL. Powder insufflator for the ear. *Otolaryngol Head Neck Surg.* 1983;91:460-461.
59. Matt BM, Miller RP, Meyers RM, et al. Incidence of perforation with Goode T Tube. *International Pediatric Otolaryngology.* 1991;21:1-6.
60. Larsen PL, Tos M, Strangerup SE. *Progression of Drum Pathology Following Secretory Otitis Media in Otitis Media.* Philadelphia, Pa: BC Decker;1988:34-38.
61. Vogelgesang MW, Birch HG. Ventilation tubes in the pediatric population. In: Lim DJ, Bluestone CD, Klein JO, Nelson J, eds. *Proceedings of the Third International Symposium: Recent Advances in Otitis Media with Effusion.* Philadelphia, Pa: BC Decker;1983;306-308.
62. Schiff M. Tympanosclerosis cause and prevention. In: Paparella MM, Meyerhoff WL, eds. Ear Clinics International. *Clinical Otology.* Baltimore, Md: Williams & Wilkins;1983;3:31-37.
63. Derlacki EL. Repair of central perforations of tympanic membrane. *Arch Otolaryngol.* 1953;58:405-420.
64. Politzer A. In: *Diseases of the Ear and Adjacent Organs.* (German trans, Cassells JP: *Lehrbuch der Ohrenheilkunde*). Philadelphia, Pa: Henry C Lea's Son and Company;1883:754.
65. Feldman WE, Ginsburg CM, McCrackin GH Jr, et al. Relation of concentration of Haemophilus influenzae type B in cerebrospinal fluid to late sequelae of patients with meningitis. *J Pediatr.* 1982;100:209-212.
66. Laxer RM, Marks MI. Pneumococcal meningitis. *Am J Dis Child.* 1977;131: 850-853.

67. Richner B, Hof E, Prader A. Hearing impairment following therapy of Haemophilus influenzae meningitis. *Helv Paediatr Acta.* 1979;34:433-447.
68. Aantaa E, Meurman OH. Meningitis in children and its effects on the action of the inner ear. *Acta Otolaryngol.* 1963;(suppl 188):145-148.
69. Keane WM, Potsic WP, Rowe LD, Konkle DF. Meningitis and hearing loss in children. *Arch Otolaryngol.* 1979;105:39-44.
70. Moss PD. Outcome of meningococcal group B meningitis. *Arch Dis Child.* 1982;57:616-621.
71. Habib RG, Girgis NI, Yassin NW, et al. Hearing impairment in mengococcal meningitis. *Scand J Infect Dis.* 1979;11:121-123.
72. Haslem RHA, Allen JR, Dorsen MM, et al. The sequelae of group B-hemolytic streptococcal meningitis in early infancy. *Am J Dis Child.* 1977;131:845-849.
73. Dodge P. Deafness in children related to meningitis; hearing loss in childhood: a primer. Columbus, OH: Ross Laboratories;1992.
74. Hib conjugate vaccines for prevention of Hib influenzae, Type B disease among infants and children 2 months of age or older. Washington, DC: Reprinted by the U.S. Department of Health and Human Services, *Public Health Service Morbidity and Mortality Weekly Report, Recommendations and Reports.* Jan 11, 1995;40,(RR-1):1-7.
75. Nadol JB. Hearing loss as a sequela of meningitis. *Laryngoscope.* 1978;88:739-755.
76. Pappas DG, Mundy MR. Sensorineunal hearing loss: infectious agents. *Laryngoscope.* 1982;92:752-754.
77. Sell SHW, Merrill RE, Doyne EO, Zimsky EP. Long-term sequelae of Haemophilus influenzae meningitis. *Pediatrics.* 1972;49:206-211.
78. Sell SHW, Webb WW, Pate JE, Doyne EO. Psychological sequelae to bacterial meningitis: two controlled studies. *Am J Dis Child.* 1975;129:212-217.
79. Rasmussen N, Johnsen N, Bohr V. Otologic sequelae after pneumococcal meningitis: a survey of 164 consecutive cases with a follow-up for 94 survivors. *Laryngoscope.* 1991;101:876-882.
80. Bluestone CD, Klein JO. Intracranial suppurative complications of otitis media and mastoiditis. In: Bluestone CD, Stool SE, eds. *Pediatric Otolaryngology.* Philadelphia, Pa: WB Saunders;1983;1:567.
81. Swartz MN, Dodge PR. Bacterial meningitis-a review of selected aspects. *N Engl J Med.* 1965;272:725–730.
82. Biggens WP, Howell NN, Newton DF, Himadi GM. Congenital ear anomalies associated with otic meningitis. *Arch Otolaryngol.* 1973;79:399-401.
83. Park TS, Hoffman HJ, Humphreys RP, Chuang SH. Spontaneous cerebrospinal fluid otorrhea in association with a congenital defect of the cochlea aqueduct and Mondini dysplasia. *Neurosurgery.* 1982;11:356-362.
84. Everland HH, Mai IW. Recurrent meningitis, congenital anacusis and Mondini anomaly. *Acta Otolaryngol (Stockh).* 1983;95:147-151.
85. Igarashi M, Schuknecht H. Pneumococci otitis media, meningitis and labyrinthitis. *Arch Otolaryngol.* 1962;76:126-130.

86. Crowe SJ. Pathologic changes in meningitis of the internal ear. *Arch Otolaryngol.* 1930;11:5.
87. Arnvig J. Relation of the ear to the subarachnoid space and absorption of the labyrinthine fluid. *Acta Otolaryngol.* 1951;(suppl 96):50-73.
88. Eavey RD, Gao YZ, Schuknecht HE, Gonzalez PM. Otologic features of bacterial meningitis of childhood. *J. Pediat.* 1985:402-406.
89. Igarashi M, Saito R, Alford BR, et al. Temporal bone findings in pneumococcal meningitis. *Arch Otolaryngol.* 1974;99:79.
90. Lebel MH, Freiz BJ, Syrogiannopoulos GA, et al. Dexamethasone therapy for bacterial meningitis. Results of two double-blind, placebo-controlled trials. *N Engl J Med.* 1988;319:964.
91. Saez-Llorens X, Ramilo O, Mustafa MM, et al. Molecular pathophysiology of bacterial meningitis. Current concepts and therapeutic implications. *J Pediatr.* 1990;116:671.
92. Mustafa MM, Ramilo O, Saez-Llorens X, et al. Cerebrospinal fluid prostaglandins, interleukin 1ß, and tumor necrosis factor in bacterial meningitis: clinical and laboratory correlations in placebo-treated and dexamethasone-treated patients. *Am J Dis Child.* 1990;144:884.
93. Committee on infectious diseases, American Academy of Pediatrics. Dexamethasone therapy for bacterial meningitis in infants and children. *Pediatrics.* 1990;86:130-133.
94. Fishman RA, Sligar K, Hake RB. Effects of leukocytes on brain metabolism in granulocytic brain edema. *Ann Neurotol.* 1977;2:289-94.
95. Baloh RW. *Dizziness, Hearing Loss, and Tinnitus: The Essentials of Neurotology.* Philadelphia, Pa: FA Davis;1984:74-94.
96. Ozdamar O, Kraus N. Auditory brainstem response in infants recovering from bacterial meningitis: neurologic assessment. *Arch Neurol.* 1983;40: 499-502.
97. Vienny H, Despland PA, Luktschg J, et al. Early diagnosis and evolution of deafness in childhood bacterial meningitis: a study using brainstem auditory evoked potentials. *Pediatrics.* 1984;73:579-586.
98. Kaplan SL, Catlin Fl, Weaver T, Feigin RD. Onset of hearing loss in children with bacterial meningitis. *Pediatrics.* 1984;73:575-578.
99. Guiscafre H, Martinex MC, Benitez-Diaz L, Munoz O. Reversible hearing loss after meningitis. Prospective assessment using auditory evoked responses. *Ann Otol Rhinol Laryngol.* 1984;93:229-232.
100. Levi-Montalcini R. Development of the acoustico-vestibular centers in chick embryo in the absence of the afferent root fibers and descending fiber tracts. *J Comp Neurol.* 1949;91:209-234.
101. Webster DB, Webster M. Mouse brainstem anditory nuclei development. *Ann Rhinol Laryngol.* 1980;89(supp 168):254-256.
102. Webster DG, Webster M. Neonatal sound deprivation affects brain stem auditory nuclei. *Arch Otolaryngol.* 1977;103:392-396.
103. Dodge PR, Davis H, Feigin RD, et al. Prospective evaluation of hearing impairment as a sequela of acute bacterial meningitis. *N Engl J Med.* 1984;311:869.

104. Ozdamar O, Kraus N, Stein L. Auditory brainstem responses in infants recovering from bacterial meningitis. Audiologic evaluation. *Arch Otolaryngol.* 1983;PD9(1):13-18.
105. Myklebust HR. *The Psychology of Deafness. Sensory Deprivation, Learning, and Adjustment.* New York: Grune & Stratton;1960;61.
106. Pappas DG, Simpson LC, Godwin, GH: Perilymphatic fistula in children with preexisting sensorineural hearing loss. *Laryngoscope.* 1988;98(No. 5):507-520.
107. Simmons FB. Sudden sensorineural hearing loss. In: Gates GA, ed. *Current Therapy in Otolaryngology-Head and Neck Surgery 1964-1985.* Philadephia, Pa: BC Decker;1984;66-72.
108. Bluestone CD, Supance JS. Perilymph fistula in infants and children. In: Gates GA, ed. *Current Therapy in Otolaryngology—Head and Neck Surgery 1984-1985.* Philadelphia, Pa: BC Decker;1984;66-67.
109. Thompson JN, Kohut RI. Perilymph fistulae: variability of symptoms and results of surgery. *Otolaryngol Head Neck Surg.* 1979;87:898-903.
110. Schulz P, Stool S. Recurrent meningitis due to a congenital fistula through the stapes footplate. *Am J Dis Child.* 1970;120:553-554.
111. Gundersen T, Haye R. Cerebrospinal otorrhea. *Arch Otol.* 1970;91:19-23.
112. Nenzelius C. On spontaneous cerebrospinal otorrhea due to congenital malformations. *Acta Otolaryngol.* 1951;4:314-328.
113. Schuknecht HF. Mondini dysplasia. A clinical and pathological study. *Ann Otol Rhinol Laryngol.* 1980;89(suppl 65):3-23.
114. Pullen FW. Round window membrane rupture: a cause of sudden deafness. *ORL.* 1972;76:1444-1450.
115. Weber P, Perez B, Bluestone C. Congenital Perilymph Fistula and Associated Middle Ear Abnormalities. *Laryngoscope.* 1993;103:160-164.
116. Nomura Y, Okuma T, Kawabata I. The round window membrane. *Adv Otolrhinolaryngol.* 1983;31:50-58.
117. Goodhill V. Leaking labyrinth lesions, deafness, tinnitus, and dizziness. *Ann Otol.* 1981;90:99-105.
118. Harada T, Sando I, Myers E. Microfissure in the oval window area. *Ann Otol.* 1981;90:174-180.
119. Weisskoff A, Murphy JT, Merzenich MM. Genesis of the round window rupture syndrome: some experimental observations. *Laryngoscope.* 1978;88: 389-397.
120. Harris I. Detection and therapy of perilymph fistulas. In: Shamhaugh GE Jr, Shea JJ, eds. *Proceedings of the Sixth Shambaugh International Workshop on Otomicrosurgery and Third Shea Fluctuant Hearing Loss Symposium.* Huntsville, Ala: Strode Publishers;1981;143-149.
121. Drake-Lee A. Immunity and graft rejection in the ear. *Immunol Today.* 1984;5:183-185.
122. Schiff M. Tympanosclerosis cause and prevention. In: Paparella M, Meyerhoff WL, eds. *Clinical Otology.* Baltimore, Md; Williams & Wilkins;1983;3:31-37.
123. McCabe BF. Autoimmune sensorineural hearing loss. *Ann Otol.* 1979;88: 585-589.

124. Hughes GB, Barna BP, Calabrese LH, et al. Immunologic disorders of the inner ear. In: Bailey BJ, ed. *Head and Neck Surgery—Otolaryngology*. Philadelphia, Pa: JB Lippincott;1993;2:1833.
125. Pappas DG, Lallone RL. Autoimmune sensorineural hearing loss. *Otolaryngology*. Ed. English GM; 1995;39(1):1-10.
126. Gussen R. Atypical ossical joint lesions in rheumatoid arthritis with sicca syndrome (Sjögren syndrome). *Arch Otolaryngol*. 1977;103:284.
127. Herberts G, Hillerdal O, Ranström S. Rhinitis, sinusitis and otitis as initial symptoms in periarteritis nodosa (Wegener's granulomatosis). *Acta Otolaryngol* (Stockh). 1966;61:189.
128. Peitersen E, Carlsen BH. Hearing impairment as the initial sign of polyarteritis nodosa. *Acta Otolaryngol*(Stockh). 1966;61:189.
129. Cogan DG. Syndrome of nonsyphilitic interstitial keratitis and vestibularauditory symtoms. *Arch Ophthalmol*. 1945;33:144.
130. Schuknecht HE. Inner ear disease in systemic (non-organ- specific) autoimmune disorders. In: *Pathology of the Ear*. 2nd ed. Philadelphia, Pa: Lea & Febiger;1993:347.
131. Yoon TH, Paparella MM, Schachern PA. Systemic vasculitis: a temporal bone histopathologic study. *Laryngoscope* 1989;99:600.
132. Veldman JE, Roord JJ, O'Connor A, Shea JJ. Autoimmunity and inner ear disorders: an immune-complex mediated sensorineural hearing loss. *Laryngoscope*. 1984;94(4):501–507.
133. McCabe B. Autoimmune inner ear disease: clinical varieties of presentation. In: Veldman JE, McCabe BF, eds. *Oto-Immunology*. Amsterdam: Kugler Publications;1987:143.

CHAPTER

6

Sensorineural Hearing Loss Associated With Trauma

*There is nothing more stimulating than a
case where everything goes against you.*
The Hound of the Baskervilles
Sherlock Holmes

BIRTH-RELATED TRAUMA

Low Birth Weight (LBW)

LBW (or prematurity), especially when accompanied by complications such as hyperbilirubinemia (which may produce jaundice) or perinatal asphyxia, is a widely accepted high risk factor for hearing loss in cases of congenitally acquired hearing impairment.[1] Other neonatal conditions that enhance the risk of neurological damage, including hearing loss, are acidosis, sepsis, presence of aminoglycoside antibiotics, incubator sound trauma, and, perhaps, hypoglycemia.[2-6] Of the foregoing, acidosis may emerge with or result from perinatal asphyxia, and the evidence indicting hypoglycemia is not conclusive. LBW rarely occurs as a solitary condition and, in itself, is seldom the cause for congenitally acquired SNHL. Determining a specific complication associated with LBW as the cause of hearing loss is difficult, if not impossible. It is possible that any one, or any combination, of these factors has a damaging effect on the auditory system.

Hyperbilirubinemia

Jaundice is probably the most commonly diagnosed pathological condition in the newborn. In 1903, Schmorl[7] defined the term "kernicterus" as jaundice of various cranial nuclear masses; today it is used clinically to apply to neurological abnormalities caused by damage to the basal parts of the brain resulting from increased bilirubin levels in the blood.

In 1932, Diamond and coworkers[8] reviewed and described the sign and symptom complex that became known as erythroblastosis fetalis, or congenital hemolytic disease of the newborn. This disorder is characterized by an abnormal retention of immature erythrocytes or erythroblasts in the bloodstream following birth and associated with edema of the fetus and jaundice. The cause of the hemolytic disease remained unknown until, in 1940, Landsteiner and Wiener[9] discovered the Rhesus factor (Rh factor), and it became obvious that this neonatal condition was due to Rh incompatibility.

Prior to the advent of the prophylactic measures now used to circumvent Rh incompatibility, kernicterus was controlled, in most cases, with exchange transfusions. Congenital hemolytic disease and its classic sequelae (including hearing impairment) were virtually eliminated by the postpartum administration of anti-D human immune globulin (Reogram) obtained from the plasma of highly sensitized Rh-negative donors. During the 1970s, it seemed that physicians clearly had the problems of neonatal jaundice under control. However, kernicterus in the absence of markedly elevated serum bilirubin levels[10] has been observed at autopsy in LBW infants. Obviously, then, other pathophysiological factors can initiate kernicterus in some neonates.

For the individual neonate, the threat of kernicterus comes to light following specific laboratory tests, such as total serum bilirubin concentration, the amount of free bilirubin,[11,12] and the reserve binding capacity (saturation) of albumin.[4] It is the unbound, or free, bilirubin that causes damage to the neurological tissue. Clinically, an empirically defined critical level of 20 or 25 mg/dl serum bilirubin constitutes a risk factor for hearing loss. The risk for kernicterus and hearing loss is not clearly defined, as the elevation in serum bilirubin level sufficient to produce hearing loss is greater in the mature infant than in the LBW neonate. However, the relationship of hyperbilirubinemia and hearing loss is most strongly revealed in LBW neonates, especially when there are concomitant conditions, such as asphyxia, acidosis, sepsis, or hypoglycemia.[3] Any one, or any combination, of these may be operative in the uptake of bilirubin by the CNS neurons. Furthermore, kernicterus has been seen in premature infants with low levels of serum bilirubin resulting from bilirubin freed from its binding with albumin by drugs (such as Gantrisin),[13] endogenously produced hematin (secondary to hemolysis), or nonesterified fatty acids[3] (NEFA) (Fig 6–1). There has been a vigorous effort made to prevent hyperbilirubinemia in neonates. New methods for the evaluation of bilirubin binding may eventually produce data useful in predicting the risk for kernicterus and hearing loss.

Perinatal Asphyxia

Asphyxia, hypoxia, and anoxia are terms used loosely to describe neonatal respiratory distress. More specifically, asphyxia is defined as impaired or absent exchange of the respiratory gases (oxygen and carbon dioxide). Hypoxia refers to the diminished availability of oxygen, and anoxia alludes to a total lack of oxygen.[15] Neither of the latter two terms, however, reflects

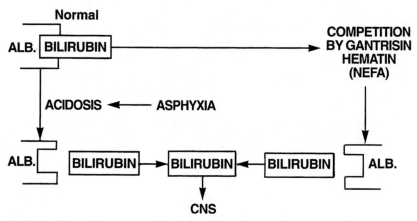

Fig 6-1.— Schematic representation of bilirubin-albumin complex separation. Unbound, or free, bilirubin represents potential CNS-diffusible bilirubin. Modified from Stern.[14] Reprinted with permission.

a specific blood content level. An early indication of partial, or incomplete, asphyxia is acidosis characterized by a decline in oxygen pressure, along with an increase in carbon dioxide, carbonic acid, hydrogen, and bicarbonic acid levels.

The causes of neonatal respiratory distress are many and include placenta previa, toxemia of pregnancy, hemorrhage, prolonged labor, cesarean and breech delivery, and a host of other conditions. The extent to which any one of these affects the CNS is difficult to assess, and for the most part, remains unclear. To facilitate recognition, the Joint Committee on Infant Hearing[1] has defined an arterial pH of less than 7.25 as a risk criterion for hearing impairment from severe asphyxia. Furthermore, the Committee states that "coma seizures or the need for assisted ventilation" in the neonate adds clinical support to the diagnosis of possible hearing loss from asphyxia. Galambos and Despland,[16] utilizing ABR testing, more specifically indicted asphyxia-related acidosis, when prolonged at birth or occurring repeatedly postnatally, as the etiological factor in their study of a group of infants manifesting impaired auditory function.

Without clinical findings supported by laboratory data, it is difficult to confirm that hearing loss results from perinatal asphyxia. Disorders of the auditory processing mechanism and certain learning disabilities associated with normal hearing that may result from perinatal asphyxia remain presumptive diagnoses whose causes have not been substantiated.

An APGAR score of less than 4 in 5 minutes, laboratory evidence of acidosis pH (less than 7.25), and clinical manifestations such as neonatal coma or seizure activity have been used as indicators of significant perinatal asphyxia. These correlations are not to be considered always factual, since it is known that SNHL can be an isolated finding, and that neonates, having suffered hypoxia, ischemia, and hemorrhagic insults will have multiple motor and/or cognitive deficits.

AUDIOMETRICS

Variations in audiometric patterns will, of course, depend on the site and degree of the original damage. Although mild-to-moderate hearing loss in the low frequencies may be indicated, bilaterally symmetrical SNHL in the high frequencies is the most common audiometric finding in cases of hearing loss secondary to hyperbilirubinemia.[17,18] Similar types of hearing loss have been found in patients whose births were complicated by asphyxia. In the author's 6-year study of 12 patients with hearing loss due to hyperbilirubinemia or asphyxia, the hearing levels have tended to remain stable, although there has been a question of mild increased threshold levels in two patients (Fig 6–2).

In addition to a hearing loss, children with damage due to kernicterus or asphyxia have clinically obvious organic disturbances resulting in various disabilities. Myklebust has stated that children with kernicterus or asphyxia act more as if they have brain damage than an impairment.[19] That is, the real difficulty in these children is not an elevated hearing threshold, but a psychoneurological disorder. In addition to the extreme disorder of cerebral palsy, lesser, but nonetheless serious,

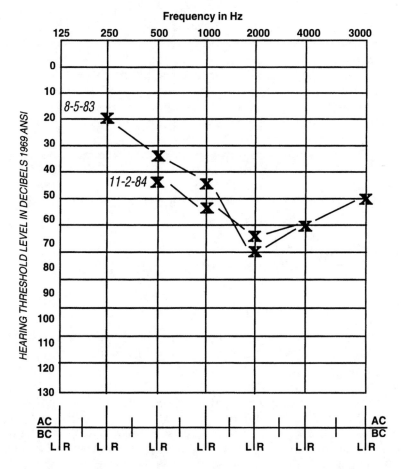

Fig 6-2.— Audiogram of a child with a moderate SNHL, presumably caused by a combination of factors (low birth weight, perinatal asphyxia with acidosis, hyperbilirubinemia). The left ear, especially, has required monitoring with audiograms since variations in hearing levels occur sporadically. This child has had amplification with hearing aids since age 2 years, has excellent speech and language at age 5 years, and has no evidence of psychoneurological-social disabilities.

conditions have been reported, including coordination problems, athetoid movements, aphasia, and a generally depressed IQ level.[20] Aphasia and hearing loss pose problems in meeting the educational needs of such children regardless of the mode of education.

PATHOPHYSIOLOGY

The damaging effects of bilirubin and asphyxia on the auditory system have been substantiated,[17,21,22] but are still unclear. Some authorities report a central auditory nucleus deafness, whereas some postulate that there is functional evidence that the lesion is peripheral,[23] others believe it is peripheral and central,[16] and still others specifically place the lesion in the cochlear nerve.[24] Nevertheless, the fact that certain nuclei in the CNS are highly susceptible to damage from increased bilirubin levels while others are damaged by anoxia,[10] either as a solitary condition or as an accompaniment, cannot be discounted.

Some of the effects seen as a result of the alteration of cells and nuclei due to increased bilirubin levels and asphyxia include swelling, hemorrhage, and degeneration.[10] In the case of bilirubin, the unbound bilirubin enters the barriers of the brain to accumulate in the cell bodies of its neurons.

HEAD INJURIES AND ACQUIRED SNHL

Temporal Bone Fracture

Auditory damage following head injury may be classified as follows: (1) hearing loss caused by longitudinal fracture of the temporal bone, (2) hearing loss caused by transverse fracture of the temporal bone, and (3) hearing loss without evidence of temporal bone fracture (labyrinthine concussion).

Injuries to the temporal bone are either longitudinal or transverse (Fig 6–3). Longitudinal fractures are caused by blows to the side of the head (temporoparietal), and the fracture usually extends from the middle ear to the region of the gasserian ganglion. Typically, the fracture lacerates the tympanic membrane and produces a steplike deformity of the external auditory canal. CSF, hemorrhagic otorrhea, and ossicular damage are common. Such an injury will cause a conductive hearing loss[25] and temporary (usually) facial nerve damage in 25% of patients. The vestibular end-organ, however, is rarely damaged.[26] In one series, which was small,

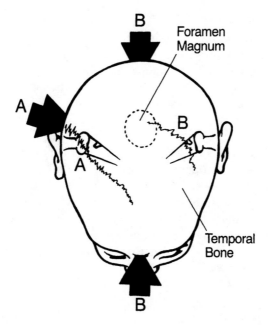

Fig 6-3.— A, Longitudinal fractures of the temporal bone result from blows to the temporoparietal area and typically cause injury to the more external structures of the ear (external canal, middle ear). B, The impact of transverse fractures is exerted over the frontal or occipital areas, causing injury to the more internal structures of the ear (auditory and vestibular nerve and their organs, facial nerve).

25 of 50 children with head injury were identified as suffering from some form of hearing loss. In this series, 16 patients had a conductive loss, and the prognosis was less certain for those who did develop a SNHL.[27]

Permanent damage to the seventh cranial nerve is uncommon in longitudinal fractures. However, transverse fractures pass through the vestibule of the inner ear, and such damage may occur from blows forceful enough to produce serious head injury with loss of consciousness. Usually, this type of injury is a result of a blow to the occipital or frontal area, with the fracture line running perpendicular across the temporal bone, originating from either the occipital bone in the area of the foramen magnum or the frontal bone. The vestibular and cochlear nerves are typically lacerated, causing an SNHL and vertigo. The facial nerve is lacerated in 50% of cases, especially at the site of the geniculate ganglion.[26] The tympanic membrane remains intact, hemotympanum is infrequent, and cerebrospinal fluid leakage is common, draining from the middle ear through the eustachian tube to the pharynx.

When the fragments of the fracture are not greatly displaced, the fracture may be impossible to demonstrate with conventional radiography, although the neurological deficits may be obvious on physical examination. However, CT tomography of the temporal bone with image enhancement techniques has been shown to diagnose fractures accurately[28] (Fig 6–4).

Bilateral SNHL has been known to occur in bilateral fractures, usually transverse, of the temporal bone. Since the skull of a small child is elastic, inward compression of the vertex surface secondary to extensive head injury may result in comminuted or extensive lines of fractures.[29] In any case, the early care of temporary bone fractures is directed toward the treatment of CSF otorrhea and facial paralysis of immediate onset. Delayed care is concerned primarily with hearing rehabilitation.[30] Meningitis is, fortunately, a rare late complication of both types of temporal bone fracture.[31]

Labyrinthine Concussion

Hearing loss, vertigo, and tinnitus often follow a head injury that does not necessarily result in a temporal bone fracture. Characteristically, this type of injury may be analogous to a brain concussion. In such an injury a disturbance of consciousness occurs with no immediate or obvious pathological change in the brain.[32] The external sites of injuries resulting in labyrinthine concussion are the areas of the temporal and occipital bones. Quite obviously, the closer the trauma is to the labyrinth, the more likely the labyrinth is to be damaged.

Audiometric evaluation of animals (cats) subjected to head blows indicated hearing lapses, particularly in the region of 4000 Hz.[33] Gross and microscopic studies of the brain and temporal bone in these animals failed to demonstrate any pathological lesions. Using graphic reconstructions of the cochlea, Schuknecht and coworkers found the site of injury to be in the upper part of the basal coil of the organ of Corti, where there was evidence of degenerative change. These investigators compared the effect of pressure waves within the organ of Corti caused by head injury to airborne blast waves or intense noise to the inner ear. In severe head injuries without evidence of temporal bone fracture, Schuknecht and colleagues also determined that increased thresholds may be found for frequencies of hearing.[33]

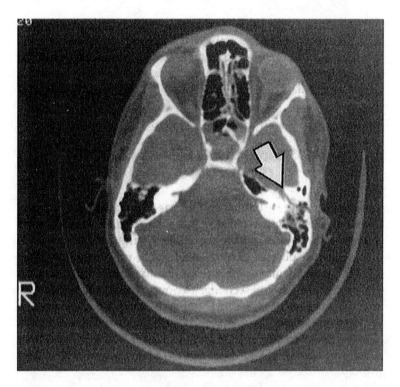

Fig 6-4.— CT scan of 19-year-old patient with longitudinal fracture of the temporal bone. The following findings are pertinent: tympanic membrane laceration, hemotympanum, conductive hearing loss, CSF otorrhea, and intact facial nerve. The fracture line originates from the outer cranial table and extends into the floor of the middle cranial fossa.

OTITIC BAROTRAUMA

Otitic barotrauma, or aerotitis, is damage to the spaces of the middle ear caused by severe negative pressure resulting from the failure of the eustachian tube to open sufficiently. Typically, otitic barotrauma occurs during rapid descent from high altitudes or rapid ascent from underwater diving. The main symptom of this condition is pain lasting for several hours. Physical evidence of the damage from this intense negative pressure may include medial displacement of the tympanic membrane, hyperemia, edema, and ecchymosis of the mucous membranes of the middle ear. Beaded extravasated blood may be seen in the tympanic membrane, especially in the area of the long process of the malleus, and fluid—at times mixed with blood—may be seen in the tympanum. A conductive hearing loss is commonly associated with this trauma. When vertigo and SNHL are associated with otitis barotrauma, a perilymph fistula has probably resulted from a tear of the window membranes.

NOISE-INDUCED HEARING LOSS (SOUND TRAUMA)

Noise is one environmental factor that has been demonstrated conclusively to cause hearing loss. Although it may be brief, daily exposure to loud noise produces a temporary hearing loss (temporary threshold shift); with continued exposure, permanent damage may result (permanent threshold shift). Difficulty with speech discrimination is a manifestation of a permanent threshold shift secondary to sound trauma. Total hearing loss is very rarely caused by excessive exposure to loud noise, however.

Factors influencing the auditory damage produced by sound trauma include the intensity of the noise and the duration of exposure. Because of individual susceptibility, the degree of damage cannot be estimated accurately. Although increased noise levels and length of exposure appear to be within the criteria established for risk of damage to an adult, there is little evidence to support the assumption that similar criteria can be used for infants.

Infant Incubator Noise Characteristics

The sound-pressure levels in incubators are reported to be approximately 57 dB to 82 dB on the linear (unweighted) scale,[5,34-37] indicating that most of the reported sound pressure levels in incubators are consistently below the adult criteria for risk of damage. The sound energy from the sources of incubator noise—the electric motor and fan— is below 500 Hz,[5] with peak sound levels obtained at 125 Hz.[37] The evidence for incubator noise as a cause of auditory damage is indirect and consists mainly of results of animal studies in which the cochleas of the younger animals sustained more damage than those in the older animals when exposed to loud sounds.[38] It has also been reported that there is a synergistic effect between the overall sound pressure level of the incubators and the potentiating effects that can occur with the combination of noise with ototoxic drugs,[6,39-41] which are frequently administered to infants in NICUs. The evidence is sufficient to warrant concern, especially since sick infants may spend 24 continuous hours in incubators for weeks at a time.

Noise Levels and Recreational Activities

Rock music, snowmobiles, model airplanes, toy guns, arcade games, and, especially, firearms have been reported to produce noise levels potentially dangerous to a child's hearing.[42-44] The factors previously mentioned (length of exposure, individual susceptibility, and so forth) that may influence damage must also be considered. The risk of noise-induced hearing loss appears minimal for most normally hearing children. However, exposure of children with SNHL to loud noises should be avoided even though the effects of loud sounds have not been studied in these children. This is especially true in light of the fact that the power output of hearing aids will intensify any sound.

The amplified sound effects of modern rock music appeal to the young. Studies indicate that the sound pressures produced by rock bands reach levels greater than 92 dB.[42,45] With this intensity of sound, the frequencies involved are commonly 500 and 800 cycles per second. These frequencies and intensities were predicted to produce as much as a 40 dB threshold shift in the area of 4000 Hz in 10% of ears exposed when sustained for a period of 1 hour. This temporary threshold shift would be expected to exceed those considered safe for prolonged exposure. Dey[46] has elucidated the effect on the auditory system of listening to tape recordings of music: After listening for 2 hours at a 100 dB sound level, 2% of individuals with hearing loss would recover, but too slowly; at 110 dB, 16% would probably sustain permanent hearing damage.

The noise of the home environment must also be considered in children receiving amplification with powerful hearing aids because of an SNHL. This includes the noise produced by a garbage disposal (80 dBA), food blenders (88 dBA), and dishwashers (75 dBA). The sound levels of a vacuum cleaner, television, and radio may reach 70 dBA[47] (Table 6–1). The background noises of a home environment may be intense enough to affect the ability of the child with hearing impairment to learn to listen.

Exposure to noise is a real concern in a child who wears hearing aids for SNHL. In the normal hearing individual, there is tremendous intersubject variability and susceptibilities to noise-induced hearing loss. Some people are sensitive, and others are not. According to Lieberman,[48] if a large group is exposed to an identical sound source, a wide range of

Table 6–1. Environmental Noises

Overall Level dBA (SPL re 0.0002 microbar)	Industrial and Military	Community or Outdoor	Home or Indoors
130	Diesel engine room (125 dB)	50 hp siren (100 ft) (125 dB)	
Uncomfortably Loud	Armored Personnel Carrier (123 dB)	Thunderclap overhead (120 dB)	
120	Oxygen torch (121 dB) Scraper-loader (117 dB) Compacter (116 dB)	Jet plane (at ramp) (117 dB)	Rock band (108-114 dB)
110	Riveting machine (110 dB) Textile loom (106 dB)	Jet flyover at 1000 ft (103 dB)	
100	Electric furnace areas (100 dB) Farm tractor (98 dB)	Power lawn mowers (96 dB) Compressor at 20 ft (94 dB) Rock drill at 100 ft (92 dB)	Inside subway car, 35 mph (95 dB)
90	Newspaper press (97 dB)	Motorcycles at 25 ft (90 dB)	Cockpit light aircraft (90 dB Shouted conversation (90 dB)
80	Cockpit-propeller aircraft dB) (88 dB)	Propeller aircraft flyover at 1000 ft (88 dB)	Food blender (88 dB)
Moderately Loud	Milling machine (85 dB)		

dB			
70	Cotton Spinning (83 dB) Lathe (81 dB)	Diesel truck, 40 MPH at 50 ft (84 dB)	Garbage disposal (80 dB) Clothes washer (78 dB)
60	Tabulating (80 dB)	Diesel train, 40-50 MPH at 100 ft (83 dB)	
50 quiet		Passenger car, 65 MPH at 25 ft (77 dB)	Living room music (76 dB)
40		Near freeway-auto traffic (64 dB)	Dishwasher (75 dB)
30 very quiet		Air conditioning unit at 20 ft (60 dB)	Vacuum (70 dB) Normal conversation (50-60 dB)
20		Large transformer at 200 ft (58 dB) Light traffic at 100 ft (50 dB)	
10 Just Audible		Rustling leaves (20 dB)	
0 Threshold of Hearing			

From JA Bell, *Physician's Guide to Noise Pollution*.[47] Reprinted with permission of American Medical Association 1973.

hearing loss results. Some people are unaffected, and others might have noise-induced hearing loss of 40-60 dB. The extent to which susceptibility is correlated with age, sex, and race is controversial. This intrasubject variability complicates the process of defining safe versus dangerous levels of sound. It is difficult to determine what damage can occur in a child with SNHL using amplification and being exposed to spurts or periods of increased noise levels, such as the trash masher in the kitchen, the blender, a lawn mower, power leaf blower, battery operated toy trucks, cars, and tools. It is advisable to remove the hearing aids or at least decrease the power levels when known exposure to certain sounds will be employed.

Noise Levels in School

The extent to which noise poses a problem in the development of speech, language, listening, and related skills is unknown.[47] The data available are not sufficient to draw any strong conclusions. Nevertheless, noise levels measured in some schools are less than ideal. Mills noted that architects pursue A-weighted sound levels of 30 to 40 dB in empty classrooms.[49] Nober[50] has reported that the average sound level of four elementary classrooms was approximately 65 dBA. According to Mills, rooms allocated as "special teacher rooms" were found to have sound levels of 40 dBA, putting them in alignment with the architectural goals.

The extent of noise levels in schools depends on many factors, such as the proximity of an institution to freeways, airports, or railways and the peak levels of noise produced by such unusually noisy vehicles as trucks, the noise of power tools in workshops, band practices, and stairway noises. Window air conditioners produce noise levels of 40 to 60 dB and, obviously, a child with hearing impairment involved in classwork should not be seated in close proximity to a functioning window air conditioner.[51]

PATHOPHYSIOLOGY OF SOUND TRAUMA

The use of the scanning electron microscope, along with the light and transmission electron microscopes, has made it possible to determine changes in the physicochemical processes of the sensory cells caused by sound trauma.[52] These changes include the formation of blebs on the surface of the hair cells, followed by vesiculation, which progresses to vacuolization of the smooth endoplasmic reticulum. Such physicochemical changes resulted in the accumulation of lysosomal granules in the subcuticular region, deformation of the cuticular plates, and, eventually, cell rupture and lysis.

Lesions produced by a 4000 Hz sound tend to produce damage near the stimulation maximum for that frequency.[53] The results from animal studies indicate existence of disagreement as to whether this damage progresses as it nears the base of tbe cochlea or whether the damage is just as great toward the apical end.[51,52]

HEARING IN THE PRESENCE OF NOISE

The infringement of environmental noise on speech intelligibility may produce a psychological effect on hearing, and disabilities may result from the decrease in hearing acuity secondary to noise-produced damage. Of course, the severity of disability a child will show will depend on the degree of damage incurred.

Background noise of sufficient intensity will reduce the perception of loudness of speech for both adults and children. However, children are probably affected more adversely since their listening skills, speech skills, and knowledge of language are less developed than those of adults. In any case, a review of the literature on the effect of noise on children[54] emphasizes that this environmental intrusion affects human performance, although some of the reports are conflicting. Normative data from this literature review, nevertheless, indicated that children require greater signal-to-noise ratios than adults to achieve the same performance level.

The Goldman-Fristoe-Woodcock[55] test of auditory discrimination shows that performance improves from about age 4 years to about age 25 years, after which it declines. The performance of children 10 years old or younger is affected more by competing noise. The significant effects of competing noise on learning in normal subjects, especially in reading skills, has been studied[56] although there may be no influence on the speed or accuracy of a performance or skill.[57]

Whether noise imposes a problem on listening skills in children and adults depends on the levels of noise found in homes, playgrounds, and schools. According to the Environmental Protection Agency's (EPA's) document of 1979, noise had a significant impact on more than 80 million people in the United States. Of that number, one half risked serious health problems from their exposure to excessive noise levels, produced primarily by automotive traffic and aircraft. Noise levels outside apartments adjacent to a busy freeway may range from 76 to 84 dBA and inside these apartments the levels may range from 52 to 70 dBA.[58,59]

SNHL ASSOCIATED WITH TOXINS

Aminoglycosides

Faced with a life-threatening sepsis, it is necessary to rely on the efficiency of some potent drugs, although the ototoxic effects of these drugs has become increasingly obvious. This is especially true in the case of infections associated with gram-negative organisms. Of the aminoglycosides used today, gentamicin (like streptomycin of earlier years) has a greater toxic effect on the vestibular system than on the cochlear system. Tobramycin sulfate and kanamycin sulfate, on the other hand, have their greatest effect on the auditory system. Hearing loss secondary to aminoglycoside ototoxicity is always sensorineural in nature, affecting primarily the high frequencies first and progressing to involve all frequencies. Profound losses have been reported with the use of some of the older ototoxic drugs.[60]

Aminoglycosides are concentrated in the perilymph and endolymph,[61] even after the drug has been discontinued and blood plasma levels have returned to normal, a characteristic not shared by other commonly used antibiotics. The ototoxicity of aminoglycosides is directly due to hair cell damage (by virtue of magnesium loss from cells that blocks enzymatic reactions)[62] and may be intensified by such associated factors as the use of other nephrotoxic drugs and defective renal or hepatic function.[63,64]

In essence, ototoxicity can be avoided in most patients with normal renal function by limiting the total dose and the length of treatment.[65] Prospective studies, using controls of large groups of neonates, have supported the low incidence of hearing loss in those treated with aminoglycosides in proper dosages.[66,67] Potential ototoxicity of aminoglycosides in infants and children was extremely small in 1300 patients studied by McCracken.[68] In monitoring patients, physicians should not dismiss the adverse effects of long-term aminoglycoside therapy and should observe such patients carefully for evidence of nephrotoxicity as well as hearing loss.

It is known that high blood levels of aminoglycosides (greater than 10 mg) are necessary for gentamycin to invade the inner ear. It would, therefore, seem logical that controlling therapeutic drug blood levels, within a margin of safety by dosage size and duration of treatment, would be the choice preventive measure.[69] Some exceptions are to be realized: (1) There is no hard core data showing that occasionally elevated peak and trough levels result in cochlear toxicity, and (2) toxicity can occur in patients whose serum levels remain within the peak trough. Matz[70] has pointed out that peak levels in some diseases have to be modified according to the nature of the infection and the pathogens. For example, for cure of endocarditis caused by resistant strain of Pseudomonas, an increased risk for toxicity is justified. On the other hand, bladder infections may be handled with lower doses that produce lower serum levels since aminoglycosides are concentrated in the urine. According to Matz, suggested schedules for determination of serum levels are as follows:

1. For patients with normal renal function, the peak level is determined within the first 1 to 2 days of therapy, the trough level within 1 week, and both peak and trough levels approximately weekly thereafter.
2. For patients with impaired but stable renal function, the peak level is determined within the first 1 to 2 days of therapy, the trough level and another peak level within 1 week, and peak and trough levels approximately twice a week from then on.
3. In the case of impaired and unstable renal function, peak and trough levels are determined within the first 1 to 2 days of therapy. Determination of serum levels may have to be made as often as daily thereafter while the renal function remains unstable.
4. After any adjustments of dosage, the peak and trough levels should be determined within 1 to 2 days.

Variances in cochlear and vestibular findings is the rule. Aminoglycoside ototoxicity may be irreversible and may even progress after the cessation of therapy. In such cases cessation of therapy may lead to improvement of inner ear function. In others, it may not. In essence, each patient receiving aminoglycoside therapy is unique and must be treated individually. The choices of testing modalities remain monitoring of renal function, serum levels, audiometric and vestibular function testing, and historical detection.

In summary, adults who have daily dosages and total dosages of aminoglycosides, as well as elevated peak-n-trough serum concentrations, have shown increased risk of ototoxicity. Audiogram studies in children and infants under 2 years of age are difficult to obtain. Nevertheless, large dosages, prolonged treatments, and decreased drug clearance, such as in patients with renal insufficiencies, have also been found to be risk factors for ototoxicity.[71,72]

Studies having to do with adults compare the ototoxicity of aminoglycosides. Kahlmeter and Dahlager,[73] having reviewed the clinical studies published between 1975 and 1982 (6494 patients), found the average incidence of cochlear toxicity to be 13.9% with Amikacin, 8% with Gentamycin, 6% with Tobramycin, and 2.4% with Netilmicin. Vestibular toxicity was studied in only 1976 patients and was found to be 3% with Gentamycin, 3.5% with Tobramycin, 2.8% with Amikacin, and 1.4% with Netilmicin.

Proof of ototoxicity from Erythromycin is lacking in children. Indeed, the first patients noted with such ototoxicity were in the Legionella pneumonia. These patients were elderly and had hepatic or renal dysfunction. The amount of Erythromycin given per day was greater than 2 grams. The ototoxicity from Vancomycin is also questionable. It has been shown in animals that Vancomycin enhances the ototoxicity of aminoglycosides.[74]

Antiprotozoal Agents

In recent years, quinine hydrochloride has been used to control leg cramps, and amebiasis has been treated with chloroquine phosphate (latter may be more of historical importance). Quinine, an abortifacient, is clinically known to produce tinnitus, hearing loss, dizziness, blurring of vision, photophobia, and hypotension[75]; the clinical side effects of chloroquine include tinnitus and imbalance.[76] Congenital SNHL from the use of both drugs has been reported.[77,78] In a study of the temporal bone of an offspring of a mother to whom chloroquine had been administered during the first trimester of her pregnancy, Matz and Naunton[77] reported that there was complete absence of hair cells and loss of many supporting cells in the organ of Corti. Degenerative changes were also found in the spiral ganglion cells of infants whose mothers had consumed high prenatal doses of quinine.

Salicylates

Light and electron microscopy have failed to reveal morphological lesions in the cochlea of animals exposed to high dosages of salicylates.[79] However, these drugs are highly concentrated in the perilymph and endolymph and produce biochemical changes in these fluids.[79] Patients receiving large dosages of aspirin complain of a high-pitched tinnitus followed by hearing loss and loss of balance. Caloric irrigations show a bilateral hypoactive response. The symptoms are dose-related and occur when plasma salicylate levels reach 0.35 mg/ml.[80] The hearing loss is characterized, in most cases, by an equal loss at all frequencies, usually at the level of 30 to 40 dB. It is completely reversible within 2 or 3 days after withdrawal of the drug.[81]

Diuretics

Ethacrynic acid and furosemide each produce a rapid-onset SNHL when given in high dosages. The hearing loss reverses within hours after the drug is discontinued. In animal studies, marked changes were demonstrated in the stria vascularis of the cochlea.[82,66]

Alcohol (Fetal Alcohol Syndrome)

Jones and colleagues, in the early 1970s,[83-85] labeled the embryonic and fetal damage resulting from the ingestion of high levels of alcohol during pregnancy as fetal alcohol syndrome (FAS). Manifestations of this condition include: (1) prenatal and postnatal growth deficiency; (2) an unusual facial pattern characterized by short palpebral fissures, epicanthic folds, mid-face hypoplasia, and a thin upper lip; (3) anomalies of joint positions and function; (4) cardiac defects; and (5) microcephaly and CNS dysfunction presenting as mental deficiency of varying degrees of severity.[86-88]

The Centers for Disease Control and Prevention reported that researchers do not know whether the present increase in FAS means improved diagnosis by doctors or whether more pregnant women are drinking. They also reported, from data compiled in 1988, that despite growing awareness that avoiding liquor prevents the syndrome, about one-fifth of women continued to drink even after they learned they were pregnant.

FAS is not a proven cause of SNHL, and its precise role in the pathogenesis of deafness is yet to be elucidated. The mental deficiency and developmental delay secondary to FAS are thought to be due to the direct toxic effect of ethanol on the developing brain. Pettigrew and Hutchinson[89] examined, by ABR, the neural function of six infants whose mothers had evidence of alcohol abuse during pregnancy. In four of these infants, evoked responses were abnormal and poorly defined, with inconsistent peaks. Threshold levels for hearing were not documented, but the results would indicate disruption of functional development of the auditory pathway in the brainstem. The results of this study are consistent with the findings and speculations of Durand and Carlen,[90] who reported depressed neuronal inhibition as a factor in impaired CNS function in ethanol-exposed animals.

Health officials do not know how much alcohol harms a fetus. Many doctors advocate no drinking at all during pregnancy, and there is evidence that even small levels of alcohol consumption can harm a fetus.

Ototoxicity From Organic Solvents and Metals

Patients often ask if certain organic solvents and/or metals are toxic to the extent that congenital hearing losses can be manifested. Organic solvents, asphyxiant gasses, and heavy metals that are present in the environment as industrial pollutants or by-products are potential hazards to the hearing mechanism. However, the real problem is the cause effect of such elements, and the lack of knowledge and research with respect to cause. The subject has been well-reviewed by Rybak,[91] who lists organic solvents that have been shown to cause hearing loss indirectly. These include trichloroethylene, xylene, styrene, hexane, carbon disulfide, toluene, carbon monoxide, butyl nitrate, and the heavy metals, which include arsenic, mercury, tin, lead, and manganese. The possibility of these elements in compounds causing congenital SNHL needs further investigation.

Others

Chemotherapeutic anticancer agents cause both auditory and vestibular ototoxicity with the main pathological findings being shrinkage of the organ of Corti.[92]

Chemotherapeutic anticancer agents such as cis-platinum are effective against a wide variety of tumors, especially embryonic lesions such as osteosarcomas, Whilm's tumors, rhabdomyosarcomas, neuroblastomas, Ewing's sarcomas, and others. This drug carries many undesirable side effects, which include ototoxicity besides that of nephrotoxicity, myelosuppression, and severe nausea and vomiting. Hearing loss has resulted with treatment of cis-platinum and involves the high frequencies, particularly that over 2000 Hz. It is progressive with continued exposure of the drug and has been shown to be most severe in children who are exposed to previous cranial radiation prior to the medication. Those who have demonstrated a hearing loss show increased deafness with successive dosing.[93]

Tobacco Fatal to Babies

Two researchers have produced startling numbers to back up the long-held belief that smoking during pregnancy can prove fatal to fetuses and infants. According to Joseph DiFranza and Robert Lew, who reviewed nearly 100 studies conducted over 40 years, mothers who smoke cause the deaths of about 5600 babies and 115000 miscarriages in the United States every year.[94]

Their study also found that mothers' smoking contributes to 53000 cases a year of LBW babies and 22000 cases of babies who require intensive care at birth.

While earlier studies have examined the risks associated with smoking during pregnancy, "no one had ever tried to calculate . . . the number of children actually harmed,"[94] said DiFranza, an associate professor of family and community medicine at the University of Massachusetts Medical Center at Worcester.

The doctors said they reached their numbers by using estimated percentages and actual numbers of how many women get pregnant each year and how many of them smoke.

The researchers[94] said that tobacco use by pregnant women results in 1900 annual cases of sudden infant death syndrome, in which apparently healthy infants are found dead in their cribs, and that an additional 3700 children died per year by the age of 1 month from complications caused by tobacco smoke during pregnancy.

HEARING LOSS AND PERSISTENT FETAL CIRCULATION[95]

Severe sloping high frequency hearing loss is typical of infants with persistent fetal circulation (PFC). The incidence of the hearing loss may be 20% or even greater, may be delayed or progressive (although it must be realized that furosemide is used in the treatment of the pulmonary condition in these studies). Besides the variable of furosemide related to those infants with confirmed hearing loss, other detrimental factors include the severity of alkalosis and the duration of the hyperventilation.

It is interesting that, although SNHL is a risk in infants with PFC, the hearing damage is not necessarily associated with overall neurologic and developmental outcomes; that is, normal cognitive abilities is the rule in PFC.

REFERENCES

1. American Academy of Pediatrics Joint Committee on Infant Hearing: Position Statement, 1982. *Pediatrics*. 1982;70:496-497.
2. Pearlman MA, Gartner LM, Lee K, et al. The association of kernicterus with bacterial infection in the newborn. *Pediatrics*. 1980;65:26-29.
3. Stern L, Doray B, Chan G, Schiff D. Bilirubin metabolism and the induction of kernicterus. *Birth Defects*. 1976;12:255-261.
4. Ballowitz L. Bilirubin encephalopathy: changing concepts. *Brain Dev*. 1980; 2:219-227.
5. Falk S, Farmer JC. Incubator noise and possible deafness. *Arch Otolaryngol*. 1973;97:385-387.
6. Bess FH, Peek BF, Chapman JJ. Further observations on noise levels in infant incubators. *Pediatrics*. 1979;63:100-106.
7. Schmorl G. Toward the understanding of jaundice in the newborn especially the theories resulting in brain changes. *Soc German Ges Pathol*. 1903;6:109-115.
8. Diamond LK, Blackfan KD, Baty JM. Erythroblastosis fetalis and its association with universal edema of the fetus, icterus gravis neonatorum and anemia of the newborn. *J Pediatr*. 1932;1:269-309.
9. Landsteiner K, Wiener AS. An agglutinable factor in human blood recognized by immune sera for Rhesus blood. *Proc Soc Exp Biol*. 1940;43:223.
10. Ahdab-Barmada M. Neonatal kernicterus: neuropathologic diagnosis in hyperbilirubinemia in the newborn. Report of the 85th Ross Conference on Pediatric Research. Columbus, Oh: Ross Laboratories; 1983:2-10.
11. Brodersen R. Prevention of kernicterus, based on recent progress in bilirubin chemistry. *Acta Pediatr Scand*. 1977;66:625-634.
12. Diamond I, Schmid R. Experimental bilirubin encephalopathy. The mode of entry of bilirubin-C into the central nervous system. *J Clin Invest*. 1966;45: 678-669.
13. Silverman WA, Anderson DH, Blanc WA, Crozier DN. A difference in mortality and incidence of kernicterus in infants allotted to two prophylactic bacterial regimes. *Pediatrics*. 1956;18:614.
14. Stern L. Bilirubin metabolism and the induction of kernicterus. *Birth Defects*. 1976;12:255-263.
15. Meyers RE. Perinatal asphyxia: Immediate and long-term effects. In: *Proceedings from the Symposia of the 5th Congress of the International Primatological Society, Nagoya, Japan, 1974*. Tokyo: Science Press, 1975.
16. Galambos R, Despland P-A. The auditory brainstem response (ABR) evaluates risk factors for hearing loss in the newborn. *Pediatr Res*. 1980;14:159-163.
17. Goodhill V. Nuclear deafness and the nerve deaf child: the importance of the Rhesus factor. *Trans Am Ophthalmol Otolaryngol*. 1950;44:671-686.
18. Crabtree N, Gerrard J. Perceptive deafness associated with severe neonatal jaundice. A report of sixteen cases. *J Laryngol Otol*. 1950;64:482-506.
19. Myklebust HR. Rh child: deaf or "aphasic"? Some psychological considerations of the Rh child . *J Speech Hear Disord*. 1956;21:423-425.

20. Vernon M. Rh Factor and deafness: the problem, its psychological, physical and educational manifestations. *Except Child*. 1967;34:5-12.
21. Dublin WA. *Fundamentals of Sensorineural Auditory Pathology*. Springfield, Il: Charles C Thomas; 1976.
22. Gerrard J. Nuclear jaundice and deafness. *J Laryngol Otol*. 1952;66:39-46.
23. Blakely RW. Erythroblastosis and perceptive hearing loss: responses of atheloids to test the cochlear function. *J Speech Hear Res*. 1959;2:5-15.
24. Chisin R, Perlman M, Sohmer H. Cochlear and brainstem responses in hearing loss following neonatal hyperbilirubinemia. *Ann Otol Rhinol Laryngol*. 1979;88:352-357.
25. Hough JVD, Stuart WD. Middle ear injuries in skull trauma. *Laryngoscope*. 1968;78:899-937.
26. Proctor B, Gurdjian ES, Webster JE. The ear in head trauma. *Laryngoscope*. 1956;66:16-59.
27. Zimmerman, WD, Ganzel, T, Windmill, N, et al. Peripheral hearing loss following head trauma in children. *Laryngoscope*. January 1993;103:87-91.
28. Shaffer KA, Haughton VM. Thin section computed tomography of the temporal bone. *Laryngoscope*. 1980;90:1099-1105.
29. Parisier SC. Injuries of the ear and temporal bone. In: Bluestone CD, Stool SE, eds. *Pediatric Otolaryngology*. Philadelphia, Pa: WB Saunders; 1983;1:614-636.
30. Cannon CR, Jahrsdoerfer RA. Temporal bone fractures. Review of 90 cases. *Arch Otolaryngol*. 1983;109:285-288.
31. Ward PH. The histopathology of auditory and vestibular disorders in head trauma. *Ann Otol Rhinol Laryngol*. 1969;78:227-238.
32. Schaller WF. After-effects of head injury. *JAMA*. 1939;113:1179-1785.
33. Schuknecht HF, Neff WD, Perlman HB. An experimental study of auditory damage following blows to the head. *Ann Otol Rhinol Laryngol*. 1951;60:273-289.
34. Falk SA, Woods NF. Hospital noise. Levels and potential health hazards. *N Engl J Med*. 1973;289:774-780.
35. Douek E, Dobson HC, Banister LH, et al. Effects of incubator noise on the cochlea of the newborn. *Lancet*. 1976;2:1110-1113.
36. League R, Parker J, Robertson M, et al. Acoustical environments in incubators and infant oxygen tents. *Prev Med*. 1972;1:231-239.
37. Seleny FL, Streczyn M. Noise characteristics in the baby compartment of incubators. *Am J Dis Child*. 1969;117:445-450.
38. Falk SA, Cook RO, Haseman JK, Sanders GM. Noise-induced inner ear damage in newborn and adult guinea pigs. *Laryngoscope*. 1974;64:444-453.
39. Jauhiainen T, Kohonen A, Jauhiainen M. Combined effect of noise and neomycin on the cochlea. *Acta Otolaryngol*. 1972;73:387-390.
40. Dayal VS, Kokshanian A, Mitchell DP. Combined effect of noise and kanamycin. *Ann Otol Rhinol Laryngol*. 1972;80:897-902.
41. Falk SA. Combined effects of noise and ototoxic drugs. *Environ Health Perspect*. 1972;2:5-22.
42. Wood BD, Bogden JD, Shapiro MJ. Elevated sound levels in New Jersey discotheques. *J Med Soc NJ*. 1979;76:661-663.

43. Axelsson A, Lindgren F. Temporary threshold shift after exposure to pop music. *Scand Audiol.* 1978;7:127-137.
44. Plakke BL. Noise levels of electronic arcade games: a potential hearing hazard to children. *Ear Hear.* 1983;4:202-203.
45. Lebo CP, Oliphant KS, Garret J. Acoustic trauma from rock-and-roll music. *Calif Med.* 1967;107:378-380.
46. Dey FL. Auditory fatigue and predicted permanent hearing defects from rock-and-roll music. *N Engl J Med.* 1970;282:467-479.
47. Bell JA. *The Physician's Guide to Noise Pollution.* Prepared for the Academy on Noise, Chicago, Il: American Medical Association; 1973.
48. Liberman, C. Loud sound: ear damage, hearing loss and ear protection. In: *Hearing Loss in Childhood: A Primer.* Columbus, Oh: Ross Laboratories; 1992: 32-38.
49. Mills JH. Noise and children: a review of literature. *J Acoust Soc Am.* 1975;58:767-777.
50. Nober LW. *A Study of Classroom Noise as a Factor Which Affects the Auditory Discrimination Performance of Primary Grade Children.* University of Massachusetts; Dissertation Abstracts International. 1973;33(A):6756. Thesis.
51. Niemoeller AF. Acoustical design of classrooms for the deaf. *Am Ann Deaf.* 1968;113:1040-1045.
52. Lim DJ, Melnick W. Acoustic damage of the cochlea. *Arch Otolaryngol.* 1971;94:294-305.
53. Stockwell CW, Ades HW, Engstrom H. Patterns of hair cell damage after intense auditory stimulation. *Ann Otol Rhinol Laryngol.* 1969;78:1144-1168.
54. Elliott DN, McGee TM. Effects of cochlear lesions upon audiograms and intensity discriminations in cats. *Ann Otol Rhinol Laryngol.* 1965;74:386.
55. Goldman R, Fristoe M, Woodcock RW. *Test of Auditory Discrimination.* Circle Pines, Mn: American Guidance Service; 1970:18.
56. Glass DC, Cohen S, Singer JE. Urban din fogs the brain. *Psychol Today.* 1973: 94-98.
57. Slater BR. Effects of noise on pupil performance. *J Ed Psychol.* 1968;59:239-243.
58. Environmental Protection Agency. *Guidance Manual for State and Local Prosecutors: Noise Violations.* Germantown, Md: Aspen Systems Corporation; 1979.
59. Cohen S, Glass DC, Singer, JE. Apartment noise, auditory discrimination and reading ability in children. *J Exp Soc Psychol.* 1973;9:407-422.
60. Nilges TC, Northern JL. Iatrogenic ototoxic hearing loss. *Ann Surg.* 1971;173: 281-289.
61. Federspil P, Schatzle W, Tiesler E. Pharmacokinetics and ototoxicity of gentamicin, tobramycin, and amikacin. *J Infect Dis.* 1976;134:S200-S205.
62. Eran D, Tamir A, Leventon G, et al. Is magnesium depletion the reason for ototoxicity caused by aminoglycosides? *Med Hypotheses.* 1983;10:353-358.
63. Ballantyne JC. Ototoxicity. In: Gibb AG, Smith MFW, eds. *Otolaryngology.* London: Butterworth Scientific; 1982;1:226-244.
64. Johnsson L-G, Hawkins JE. Symposium on basic ear research. II: strial atrophy in clinical and experimental deafness. *Laryngoscope.* 1972;82:1105-1125.

65. Wërsall J, Lundquist P-G, Bjorkroth B. Ototoxicity of gentamicin. *J Infect Dis.* 1969;119:410-416.
66. Finitzo-H-T, McCracken GH, Roeser RJ, et al. Ototoxicity in neonates treated with gentamicin and kanamycin: results of a four-year controlled follow-up study. *Pediatrics.* 1979;63:443-450.
67. Eichenwald HF. Some observations on dosage and toxicity of kanamycin in premature and full-term infants. *Ann NY Acad Sci.* 1966;132:984-991.
68. McCracken GH. Aminoglycoside toxicity in infants and children. *Am J Med.* 1986;80(6b):172-178.
69. Quick CA. Chemical and drug effects on the inner ear. In: Paparella MM, Shumrick DD, eds. *Otolaryngology.* Philadelphia, Pa: WB Saunders; 1973;2: 397-406.
70. Matz GJ. Aminoglycoside cochlear ototoxicity. In: Rybak LP, ed. *The Otolaryngol Clin NA.* October 1993;26(5):705-712.
71. Assael BM, Parini R, Rusconi F. Ototoxicity of aminoglycoside antibiotics in infants and children. *Pediatr Infect Dis.* 1982;1:357.
72. Siegel JD, McCracken GH. Aminoglycoside ototoxicity in children. In: Lerner SA, Matz, GJ, Hawkins JF, eds. *Aminoglycoside Ototoxicity.* Boston: Little, Brown & Co; 1981:341-353.
73. Kahlmeter G, Dahlager JI. Aminoglycoside toxicity: a review of clinical studies published between 1975 and 1982. *J Antimicrobrial Chemotherapy.* 1984; 13(suppl A):9-22.
74. Brummett RE. Ototoxicity of vancomycin. *The Otolaryngol Clin NA.* Rybak LP, ed. October 1993;26(5):821-828.
75. Hart CW, Naunton RF. The ototoxicity of chloroquine phosphate. *Arch Otolaryngol.* 1964;80:407-412.
76. Hennebert D, Fernandez C. Ototoxicity of quinine in experimental animals. *Arch Otolaryngol.* 1959;70:321-333.
77. Matz G, Naunton RF. Ototoxicity of chloroquine. *Arch Otolaryngol.* 1968;88: 370-372.
78. McKinna AJ. Quinine induced hypoplasia of the optic nerve. *Canad J Ophthalmol.* 1966;1:261-266.
79. Silverstein H , Bernstein JM, Davies DG. Salicylate ototoxicity. *Ann Otol Rhinol Laryngol.* 1967;76:118-128.
80. Baloh RW. *Dizziness, Hearing Loss and Tinnitus: The Essentials of Neurotology.* Philadelphia, Pa: FA Davis; 1984:149.
81. Myers EN, Bernstein JM, Fostiropolous G. Salicylate ototoxicity. *N Engl J Med.* 1965;273:587-590.
82. Quick CA, Duvall AJ. Early changes in the cochlear duct from ethacrynic acid: an electronmicroscopic evaluation. *Laryngoscope.* 1970;60:954-965.
83. Jones KL, Smith DW, Ulleland CN, Steissguth AP. Pattern of malformation in offspring of chronic alcoholic mothers. *Lancet.* 1973;1:1267-1271.
84. Jones KL, Smith DW. Recognition of the fetal alcohol syndrome in early infancy. *Lancet.* 1973;2:999-1001.

85. Jones KL, Smith DW. The fetal alcohol syndrome. *Teratology.* 1975;12:1-10.
86. Streissguth AP, Herman CS, Smith DW. Intelligence, behavior, and dysmorphogenesis in the fetal alcohol syndrome: a report on 20 patients. *J Pediatr.* 1978;92:363-367.
87. Clarren SK, Alvord EC Jr, Sumi SM, et al. Brain malformations related to prenatal exposure in ethanol. *J Pediatr.* 1976;92:64-67.
88. Shaywitz SE, Cohen DJ, Shaywitz BA. Behavior and learning difficulties in children of normal intelligence born to alcoholic mothers. *J Pediatr.* 1980;96:978-982.
89. Pettigrew AG, Hutchinson I. Effects of alcohol on functional development of the auditory pathway in the brainstem of infants and chick embryos. *Ciba Found Symp.* 1984;105:26-46.
90. Durand D, Carlen PL. Decreased neuronal inhibition in vitro after long-term administration of ethanol. *Science.* 1984;224:1359-1361.
91. Rybak L. Hearing: the effects of chemicals. *Otolaryngology, Head and Neck Surg.* 1992;106:677-686.
92. Schuknecht H. The pathology of several disorders of the inner ear which cause vertigo. *South Med J.* 1964;57:1161-1167.
93. Weatherly R, Owens J, Catlin F, Mahoney D. Cis-platinum ototoxicity in children. *Laryngoscope.* September 1991;101:917-924.
94. DiFranza J, Lew, R. Affect of maternal cigarettes on pregnancy complications in sudden death syndrome. *J Fam Pract.* April 1995;40(No 4):385-394.
95. Naulty CM, Weis IP, Herer GR. Progressive sensorineural hearing loss in survivors of persistent fetal circulation. *Ear Hear.* 1986;7:74-77.

CHAPTER

7

Basic Audiologic Evaluation of Congenital Hearing Loss

Lynn Carmichael, MSC, CCC-A, F-AAA
Michel B. Manning, MS, CCC-A

*The world is full of obvious things which
nobody by any chance ever observes.*
The Hound of the Baskervilles
Sherlock Holmes

To facilitate optimal language development in children who are hearing-impaired, the acquisition of receptive language must be initiated early, preferably by age 4 months, but no later than age 8 months. By age 18 months, normally hearing children are speaking intelligibly either in single words or two-word utterances. Success in habilitating and educating any child who is hearing-impaired is dependent on early diagnosis and therapy. Therefore, it is imperative for the family physician, pediatrician, otolaryngologist, and, most especially, the parents to exhibit a high index of suspicion regarding hearing loss.

Screening questionnaires, such as the High Risk Registry (Table 7–1),[1] and objective tests, such as ABR, may identify hearing impairment by 3 months of age. That is, children indicated to be at risk for severe to profound hearing loss by these procedures are reexamined with objective audiometry and, at the age of 3 months, the hearing loss is confirmed. Children not suspected at birth of having severe to profound hearing loss require discerning consideration of the data gathered from the historical examination, especially in the 6- to 8-month age group. The accuracy and completeness of the examiner's historical examination are of paramount importance. Typically, infants with severe to profound hearing loss will babble until approximately age 6 months. After this age, due to the absence of a hearing feedback system, this vocal play ceases. The infant who is hearing-impaired becomes silent, and the parents notice that the child does not respond to loud sounds. A history of these subjective observations is sufficient to suggest loss of hearing acuity in this age group and, strategically, the primary care physician is in a position to identify this risk factor.

Table 7–1. High Risk Registry (Indicators for Hearing Loss)

1. Family history of hereditary childhood sensorineural hearing loss.

2. In utero infection, such as cytomegalovirus, rubella, syphilis, herpes, and toxoplasmosis.

3. Craniofacial anomalies, including those with morphological abnormalities of the pinna and ear canal.

4. Birth weight less than 1500 grams (3.3 lbs).

5. Hyperbilirubinemia at a serum level requiring exchange transfusion.

6. Ototoxic medications, including but not limited to the aminoglycosides, used in multiple courses or in combination with loop diuretics.

7. Bacterial meningitis.

8. Apgar scores of 0 to 4 at 1 minute or 0 to 6 at 5 minutes.

9. Mechanical ventilation lasting 5 days or longer.

10. Stigmata or other findings associated with a syndrome known to include a sensorineural and/or conductive hearing loss.

From American Academy of Pediatrics Joint Committee on Infant Hearing: Position Statement, 1994.

Mild and moderate hearing loss cannot be easily identified in infancy or early childhood unless positive findings from the High Risk Registry lead to evaluation by objective audiometry. The stimuli of objective screening tests are too intense to identify mild to moderate hearing loss and, historically, infants with losses of these degrees engage in vocal play as do normally hearing children. Fortunately, children with this type of hearing impairment usually develop speech and language in adequate fashion. Identification of a mild to moderate hearing loss is made by obvious speech defects, usually at ages 3 to 5 years.

This chapter reviews (superficially, since so much material is available in the current literature) pure tone audiometry, infant screening, and amplification in infants and children.

PURE TONE AUDIOMETRY

Pure tone thresholds are determined by a combination of frequency and intensity. A national standard (American National Standards Institute [ANSI]) is used to quantify the degree, or amount, of hearing loss.[2] The levels of normal hearing approximate the softest sound (pure tone) that can be heard by normally hearing individuals. Hearing threshold is the difference between the normal standard for hearing and the patient's reported hearing levels.

Pure tones of selected frequencies are presented through earphones to assess air conduction thresholds and by a vibrator placed on the mastoid to determine bone conduction thresholds. The results of air and bone conduction tests are then plotted on an audiogram from which the degree (in dB) and configuration (or pattern) of the hearing loss can be determined.

Three types of hearing loss can be determined from the audiogram: conductive, sensorineural, or mixed. With a conductive hearing loss, air conduction responses are poorer than those of bone conduction. The difference in the thresholds of air and bone conduction is known as an air-bone gap. When measuring bone conduction responses, it is important to introduce a noise into the nontest ear to eliminate crossover threshold responses. The introduction of noise into the nontest ear is known as masking. Proper masking serves to give a more accurate impression of inner ear function of the test ear.

A SNHL results in an equal reduction in air and bone conduction thresholds. A mixed hearing loss is a combination of conductive and sensorineural components.

BEHAVIORAL OBSERVATION AUDIOMETRY

Normal hearing and developmental delays can be determined in early infancy with adequate pediatric audiological testing. Behavioral testing can provide information concerning not only hearing acuity, but also visual tracking and gross motor development. Parents observing behavioral testing will better understand their child's hearing acuity.

Calibrated pure tone stimulation, noise, and speech signals are used to elicit a response. The controlled test environment is a large sound-treated room in which the infant is seated in a high chair or on the mother's lap and there is adequate space for the examiner to maneuver. While an audiologist presents the sound stimuli, a pediatric audiologist observes the responses of the infant.

VISUAL REINFORCEMENT AUDIOMETRY

The hearing of children from the age of approximately 9 to 24 months, and occasionally younger, is tested by visual reinforcement audiometry. This method of testing a child's hearing offers the advantages of reinforcing the response to the sound, decreasing the effects of response habituation, and increasing the examiner's control of the child's response.[3] The calibrated sound stimulus is reinforced with either a blinking light or an animated toy that is located above the speaker through which the stimulus is presented.

PLAY AUDIOMETRY

Play audiometry involves a play activity, such as a group of pictures or a pegboard, to reinforce the calibrated sound stimulus. The 2- to 4-year-old patient is told to listen and to point to the appropriate picture or insert a peg into the board at the sound of a tone. Thus, the child is reinforced for listening. By using this method of testing, both air- and bone-conduction thresholds may be obtained.

Much of what can be achieved through any method of testing depends on the flexibility and creativity of the audiologist and the maturity of the child. By 3 years of age, many children can be tested by conventional pure tone methods.

IMPEDANCE AUDIOMETRY

Impedance is defined as the resistance of a given system (the middle ear) to a flow of energy (sound).[4] Information regarding the function of the organ of hearing has been gained by measurements of the acoustic impedance of the ear. This is a rapid, reproducible procedure that, so long as the child is cooperative, has the additional advantage of objectivity, since the information provided is not influenced by the patient's motivation, judgment, or active participation.

Acoustic compliance is the counterpart of acoustic impedance. That is, it implies ease of movement (mobility) rather than resistance (stiffness). Impedance (stiffness) or compliance (mobility) can be measured by determining the effect of air pressure introduced into the external auditory canal on the movement of the tympanic membrane.

A successfully administered impedance battery should yield three measurements for each ear: type of tympanogram, maximum static compliance, and acoustic reflex threshold (contraction of the stapedius muscle in response to loud sound).

TYMPANOMETRY AND STATIC COMPLIANCE

Tympanometry is used widely to evaluate the ability of the tympanic membrane to move in or out when the external auditory canal is patent. It is used to reinforce the otological examination, to study the function of the eustachian tube, and to give diagnostic information, such as presence of middle ear pressure aberrations from fluid or tubal occlusion, as seen in conductive hearing loss.

Plotting of compliance change is nothing more than locating the point at which middle ear pressure equals the air pressure in the external auditory canal (Fig 7–1).

A graph is made while introducing air at a positive pressure (+200 mm H_2O) and then decreasing the pressure to –500 mm H_2O. In the presence of a normal middle ear system, compliance will change as the pressure changes. The graph will form a peak, resembling a tepee, at the point where the middle ear pressure equals the external canal pressure. The peak represents the point of compliance. If the eustachian tube is partially obstructed, negative pressure occurs in the middle ear and the peak shifts to the left (minus) side of zero (Fig 7–1, 3). If movement of the tympanic membrane is prevented by the presence of fluid in the middle ear, there is no peak and the tympanogram is said to be flat (no change in middle ear compliance when the air pressure is varied in the external ear canal) (Fig 7–1, 2).

Another abnormal finding commonly identified by this procedure is the restricted tympanogram (Fig 7–1, 5). This indicates, by a reduced peak, normal middle ear pressure with limited compliance and represents a limitation in the movement of the tympanic membrane. This is

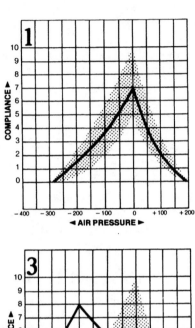

Fig 7-1.— Five characteristic tympanograms. 1. Normal, classified as Jerger Type A; 2. Flat, classified as Jerger Type B; 3. Negative presure, classified as Jerger Type C; 4. Hypermobile, classified as Jerger Type Ad; 5. Restricted, classified as Jerger Type As.

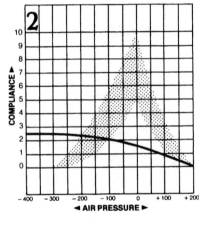

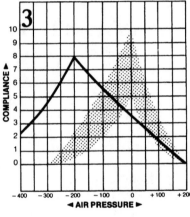

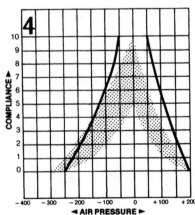

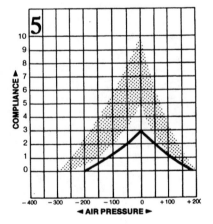

typically seen in cases of inactive chronic ear inflammation (tympanic membrane fibrosis and tympanosclerosis), congenital malleus head fixation, and otosclerosis. The converse of this situation is hypermobility of the tympanogram, which indicates a flaccid tympanic membrane (probably due to chronic eustachian tube obstruction) or a discontinuity of the ossicular chain (Fig 7–1, 4).

ACOUSTIC REFLEX

As noted earlier, acoustic reflex thresholds are determined by the contraction of the stapedius muscle in response to loud sound. Such a contraction results in a stiffening of the tympanic membrane, regardless of which ear is being stimulated by the sound. Measurement of this increased acoustic impedance (stiffness) is monitored while a loud sound is introduced into either ear. In a normally hearing subject, the acoustic reflex will be elicited when a pure tone is presented between 70 and 100 dB above hearing level.

In basic audiology, the acoustic reflex, analogous to a loudness recruitment test, is used primarily to establish the presence of a pure SNHL due to a cochlear lesion. Furthermore, a conductive hearing loss, even with an air-bone gap as small as 5 dB, will often obscure the acoustic reflex because the lesion prevents a change in compliance—that is, a change in the amount of acoustic energy reflected from the tympanic membrane. Therefore, when used with tympanometry, an absent acoustic reflex can confirm the presence of a conductive lesion. In more sophisticated audiology, the use of both crossed (contralateral) and uncrossed (ipsilateral) acoustic reflexes offers differential diagnostic information for the site of an auditory lesion.

AUDITORY BRAINSTEM RESPONSE (ABR)

With the use of averaging computers, it is possible to compile and analyze evoked electrical potentials that arise from the auditory nerve system. To record these potentials, electrodes are attached to the vertex and mastoid areas, and repetitive sounds are presented to the ear.

The absolute latency of the ABR waveforms depends on the intensity of the stimulus.[5] Threshold levels are identified by decreasing stimuli from high (loud) levels to low (soft) levels (Fig 7–2). Combined techniques are necessary to approximate the entire pure tone audiogram. Click stimuli produce stimuli in the mid to high frequency (1500-4000 Hz)

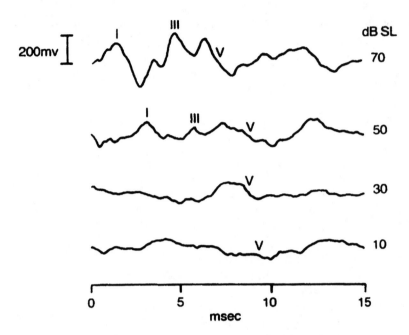

Fig 7-2.— ABR of an infant with normal hearing induced by clicks of varying intensity levels (70–10 dB). In determining threshold hearing, each ear is first tested at level of 70 dB. A judgment is made as to whether or not Wave V is present. If not, the intensity level is increased to 80 dB and, if necessary, to 90 dB. The scale at the bottom of the figure identifies the latency of the wave peaks. If Wave V is identified at 70 dB, with a latency between 7 and 11 msec, trials are initiated at 50, 30, and 10 dB sound level to confirm the presence of normal hearing. Typically, Wave V in normal infants will show smaller amplitudes and slightly longer latencies as the sound levels is decreased.

range, while tone bursts (usually 500 Hz) are used to obtain low frequency information.

SCREENING STRATEGIES FOR IDENTIFICATION OF HEARING LOSS

Hearing screening is a method of detecting hearing impairment prior to the time that it becomes obvious. Programs and procedures for screening newborn hearing have been modified and improved in the past few years.[6,7] Clearly, the screening procedure for any disorder is a task that can be accomplished rapidly, accurately, economically, and with little energy or resources misspent pursuing the so-called normals. No diagnostic screening device fully fills these criteria.

The incidence of hearing loss is not rare and when the loss is identified, it is of no little consequence. Hearing loss occurs in 1 of 50 to 56 infants[8,9] in the NICU and 1 in 700 to 200[10-12] in the well-baby nursery. The following diagnostic methods focus on the viable means of detecting hearing loss in neonates.

Objective Hearing Screening Strategies

Acoustic Reflex and Neonatal Screening

Because of the presence of middle ear effusion in infants and the lack of maturity of the acoustic reflex in the neonate, normal acoustic reflex thresholds cannot be considered an accurate screening procedure.

Automated ABR

In the screening of hearing acuity in neonates, the most commonly used procedure is automated ABR. With automated ABR, a series of clicks are presented while the infant is sleeping. Waveforms are recorded and compared to the responses of normal hearing infants. If the response matches the norms, the infant passes. If the responses do not match, the infant is referred for further testing. If a hearing loss is indicated by ABR screening, testing should be repeated in 3 to 4 months,[13] at which time the test results should supply unequivocal evidence for or against a peripheral hearing disorder.

Otoacoustic Emissions

Otoacoustic emissions (OAEs) may be simply defined as low-level sounds generated by the cochlea and measurable in the external auditory canal. This procedure is noninvasive and involves the insertion of a probe tip into the ear canal to present a stimulus which can elicit a response from the outer hair cells of the cochlea. This procedure has the advantage of being rapid, reproducible, and objective—requiring no active participation from the patient. For these reasons, OAEs are considered especially beneficial for infants and persons with multiple disabilities.

Although evoked OAEs cannot give a clear picture of the degree of hearing loss, the presence of OAEs within established norms indicates hearing within normal limits. In contrast, an absence or reduced presence of OAEs is an indication of hearing loss.

Utility of Methods

All deficits in the hearing acuity of neonates indicated by objective screening methods must be retested in 3 months by ABR or behavioral audiometry to differentiate them from permanent hearing losses. There is no true advantage in attempting to confirm the presence of hearing loss prior to hospital discharge. That is, there is nothing to gain in supplementing one screening method by another during the neonatal period.

Cost must be addressed, especially when a well-baby nursery[14] is involved, for only 1 infant in 700 to 2000 in a well-baby nursery may be identified as having a hearing loss. However, should that one child not be identified until the age of 2 to 3 years, the cost in terms of habilitation, education, psychosocial stigmata, and potential employment opportunities as an adult are insurmountable. On the other hand, if a hearing loss is identified at birth, early habilitation may diminish its effects to the extent that the child may have every opportunity to fully develop to his or her potential. For this reason, early screening programs are an essential route to acquisition of speech and language.

Study To Confirm Hearing Loss

The effectiveness of a program to screen hearing is dependent on well-coordinated follow-up. When a neonate fails the hearing screening, complete audiological testing is recommended by age 3 months to confirm the presence or absence of hearing loss.

Either the parents or the testing institution must take responsibility for the follow-up examination. The pediatrician or primary care physician must be alerted when a hearing loss has been identified. The parents and physicians must be aware of the significance of hearing loss and the efforts needed to compensate for and habilitate the hearing loss. This effort will be shared among the physician, parents, and the appropriate educators. This would involve specific educational efforts and the hiring of competent personnel to coordinate the child's habilitation program.[15]

History Examination for Screening

There are several factors that make early identification of SNHL difficult. Mild to moderate hearing loss may be missed by screening procedures. Also, hearing loss may be acquired following birth, and some infants with delayed hereditary SNHL hear normally at birth but develop a hearing loss during the first year of life. The present strategy of screening for hearing loss in children is based on age and is applied either at birth or when the child enters a preschool or public school system. The ages from 3 months to 3 or 4 years have not been a target for objective screening, although screening questionnaires may be effective.

AMPLIFICATION STRATEGY FOR HEARING IMPROVEMENT

An integral part of any comprehensive habilitation program for a child with SNHL is appropriate binaural amplification. There is an abundance of documented information evaluating the various methods of amplification with statistics reflecting their use, and this information will not be reiterated here.

Some principles of amplification and their variables will be highlighted in this section. Interspersed with these are descriptions of the problems encountered with amplification and clinical proposals to elucidate them.

Hearing Aids and Residual Hearing

Infants can be fit with hearing aids as soon as the hearing loss is confirmed, even prior to age 3 months. Many factors, including individual differences, influence the extent and nature of successful amplification. However, even children with profound hearing loss can benefit from the use of hearing aids. It is common knowledge among professionals that some children with profound SNHL learn speech and develop language, whereas others do not. In addition to early factors, identification of the hearing loss and appropriate education at an early age, binaural amplification fosters the best possible adjustment to a hearing disability. Attention to these early factors[16] (identification, binaural amplification, and education) does not necessarily ensure, but certainly facilitates, the acquisition of speech and language by the child with profound hearing loss. The task of speech and language development is benefitted by appropriate amplification. Children exposed to these benefits become aware of sound, develop localization and discrimination of sound, and learn to monitor their voices. These supplementary skills augment functional speech perception to enhance the benefits of an auditory or oral program and promote emerging skills in total communication.

There is a small percentage (1% or less) of children who have bilateral total hearing loss (ECHO statistics of 400 children evaluated). In some children diagnosed as having total hearing loss in infancy, residual hearing may emerge by age 6 months to 1 year through enhanced auditory experience.[17] In those children who reach the age of 1 to 2 years without adequate aided responses, the cochlear implant may be a viable option.

Exploitation of Residual Hearing

In some pediatric SNHL patients, residual hearing is not being utilized to its greatest potential. Over one half of a group of 100 aided children who were referred to the Pappas ECHO Foundation were found to have inadequate amplification. That is, both children with moderate to severe and profound hearing loss could not detect sounds in the "speech banana." It should not be assumed that a child wearing a hearing aid can "hear." Residual hearing must be used effectively. If this is not achieved, the intent of amplification is not being fully realized and faulty amplification must be strongly suspected.

Furthermore, in many of the Pappas ECHO Foundation cases, too much valuable early time was expended before the hearing loss was identified and aided. Hearing thresholds are identifiable at any age and time. If there is a question regarding hearing acuity, the child should be referred to a pediatric audiologist with experience in identifying and habilitating hearing loss in children.

Early Amplification

The use of binaural hearing aids for amplification in children who are hearing-impaired is no longer controversial.[18] The choice of binaural amplification is based on several factors,[19-22] the key ones being the following: (1) listening with both ears has been shown to be advantageous when listening in the presence of noise; (2) binaural summation provided by the use of two hearing aids results in an additional 3 dB of loudness; (3) binaural amplification produces an 8 to 24% increase in discrimination ability; and (4) localization skills can be developed with the use of two hearing aids. To these advantages can be added a psychosocial benefit: at any time one third to one half of the hearing aids in use by children are either nonfunctional or malfunctioning enough to significantly distort sound,[23-25] during which time the opposite aid gives functional amplification.

Mild and Moderate Hearing Losses

Over the past decade, mild and moderate hearing loss in children has received a large amount of attention. The primary reasons for this are as follows: (1) the heightened awareness for amplification to facilitate speech and language development, and (2) the demonstration that such hearing losses may progress to more severe levels.

Guidelines for amplification in children differ from those in adults. It has been demonstrated that even mild hearing loss can have an impact on the development of speech and oral language. Therefore, any approach to hearing aid assessment in young children must consider the speech, language, and vocal factors in a systematic manner. Children having minimal hearing loss must be evaluated individually according to speech defects, specific language disorders, and academic performance.

Most cases of mild and moderate SNHL are diagnosed late or in older children, usually after age 3 years (statistics from the Pappas ECHO Foundation). It has been reported that approximately 50% of all children with SNHL in the 26 to 45 dB range do not consistently use hearing aids.[26-28]

Progression of hearing loss may be expected in cases of viral and infectious diseases, as well as delayed inherited hearing losses. Early identification, intense audiological monitoring, and prompt habilitation are essential in cases of progressive hearing loss.

Speech Spectrum

The principle of the "speech spectrum" must be considered in the auditory process of normal and aided hearing. These sensitivity curves of normal human hearing permit an audiogram of an individual with hearing impairment to be directly compared to the levels shown.[29]

Children with hearing impairment who have appropriate amplification can detect most sounds in the speech frequencies of 30 to 50 dB.[30] Through auditory training, children with SNHL learn to develop their listening skills to listen for very soft sounds. Ling and Ling[31] have reported that a child who has residual hearing through 1000 Hz should be able to detect the majority of consonant sounds.

In addition to its primary function of speech detection, other spectral information may be obtained by bringing amplified hearing into the speech spectrum. Frequency, intensity, and duration of sound are nonlinguistic elements of speech that provide acoustic information. To have control of the suprasegmental aspects of speech, amplification must reach the speech spectrum. The speech spectrum can provide a basic tool for the physician or clinician in assessing the need for amplification in the child with a minimal or mild hearing loss. Should a mild SNHL be diagnosed in the infant-child years, the use of the speech spectrum may better demonstrate the phonetic implications of the hearing impairment. In the older child with mild SNHL, the decision to use amplification is based on a review of audiological findings, phonetic implications from the speech spectrum, consideration of the child's progress in speech and language development, and evaluation of school performance.

Monitoring the Child With Hearing Aids

Changes in hearing performance are commonly seen in children using hearing aids due to a SNHL. The causes for these changes include malfunctioning hearing aids,[31,32] SOM, additional acquired causes such as meningitis, progression of the hearing loss due to continued existence of causative factors, and possibly sound trauma from a hearing aid, itself. These conditions are discussed elsewhere in this book.

Failure to monitor the hearing levels more than once a year is negligence. Notwithstanding the possibility of preventing or effectively treating the cause of progression in the hearing loss and averting potential damage, a worsening of thresholds over a period of 12 months in children with mild to severe hearing loss may change amplified levels from those consistent with "hearing" to those representing "hearing-impaired." That is, a mere shift of 15 dB in hearing may mean the difference between hearing and not hearing speech. Personnel in educational programs must be in a position to detect changes in hearing thresholds if adequate amplification is to be provided. It is also important that parents and educators recognize changes in aided hearing performance. Subjectively, this can be done by using the spoken voice symbols of Ling and Ling.[33] Objectively, hearing should be monitored with unaided and aided audiograms every 3 months for the first year following identification of the hearing loss. During periods when the hearing is unstable, weekly audiograms are recommended. If the hearing remains stable, then hearing should be monitored every 6 months until age 8 years. At age 8 years or older, hearing should be monitored annually. In all cases, children should be examined whenever a change in speech performance is noticed by the parents or educators.

Hearing Aid Assessment

The performance of the hearing aid may be evaluated in several ways. In the adult, a hearing aid is well fit when it allows the person to monitor the speaking voice so that good quality and good speech timing may be achieved. However, such characteristics cannot be evaluated in the child who is hearing-impaired who has little or no speech.

The following assessments of hearing aid function should be made:

▶ Soundfield aided audiogram
▶ Hearing aid electroacoustic analysis
▶ Real ear measurement (REM)
▶ Observation

The soundfield aided audiogram examines the subject, the hearing aid, and the earmold. As previously discussed, reexamination by soundfield aided audiogram varies according to the hearing needs of the child. Due to limited expressive language skills in young children, discrimination scores usually cannot be elicited. This is especially true in the presence of severe to profound hearing loss. In the child who is hearing-impaired, aided test scores confirm the hearing aid function needed to hear speech sounds. Aided audiograms, as well as residual hearing thresholds, must be monitored.

Electroacoustic analysis of hearing aids measures hearing aid output performance as well as distortion. Other information provided by the hearing aid analyzer is frequency response and the level of gain at each frequency.

REMs are an effective tool for determining how well a hearing aid is serving an individual's hearing loss. This test involves carefully inserting a probe tube into the ear canal after the audiological thresholds of each ear have been entered into the computer. A stimulus of 200 to 8000 Hz is then presented to provide the audiologist with the real ear unaided response curve. A fitting formula is then selected and, with the probe tube still in place, the hearing aid is inserted into the ear. The stimulus is presented, which provides the tester with the real ear aided response curve. These results provide information regarding the amount of amplification provided at individual frequencies.

Observation by the educator and parents is indispensable in monitoring the hearing acuity of a child who is hearing-impaired and the function of his or her hearing aid. The use of Ling and Ling's five sound test[34] can provide information about the detection and discrimination of various sounds. Also, a change in the hearing-learning performance of the child may be striking, even with a 10 to 15 dB decrease in hearing acuity. If a difference in hearing and listening ability is detected, it is necessary to test unaided and aided hearing, analyze the hearing aids, and examine for middle ear pathology.

Frequency Modulation (FM) Systems

The amplification system typically found in a educational setting is the FM system. The modern FM systems are essentially binaural hearing aids with the addition of frequency-modulated transmission of radio frequency (RF). The RF system is very similar to the usual FM radio system, as it incorporates a microphone and a transmitter for the teacher and a receiver for the pupil. The signal is picked up by the receiver and converted back into acoustic energy. The most important function of the unit is to deliver the words of the teacher at a favorable signal-to-noise (S/N) ratio.

Environmental microphones also allow the unit to serve as personal hearing aids when the FM signal is switched off. This versatility permits the reduction of signal-to-noise ratio, allows distance hearing, and makes possible the listening skills necessary in everyday life.

There are currently several manufacturers offering a combination hearing aid behind-the-ear (BTE)-FM hearing system. These devices enable high quality FM signals to be received directly at ear level by utilizing an integrated BTE/FM receiver hearing aid approximately the size of other BTE hearing aids.

Hearing Aid Sound Trauma

The data thought to demonstrate decreased hearing sensitivity from use of high-powered hearing aids by pediatric patients were examined and found to be hasty generalizations.[35-45] Well-documented medically and scientifically adequate case studies implicating trauma from hearing aids are few and reflect only a small percentage (approximately 0.2%) of the total reported pediatric population with hearing impairment. A fundamental reason for rejecting claims of acoustic over-amplification as the determinant of deteriorating hearing among children includes the progressive nature of the hearing loss of both congenital and acquired types. Over-amplification may be a contributing factor or indirect cause in some cases of progressive hearing loss. The need to provide more detailed and controlled case studies is obvious.

Prescription of powerful hearing aids should be done professionally for each individual patient. There is no doubt that meticulous care should be taken in monitoring children using high gain instruments. If an increase in high frequency gain is deemed necessary due to failure to reach the speech spectrum, the audiologist must closely monitor the hearing when the maximum power output is increased above 128 dB. Attaining speech and language through audition becomes a more important factor than fear of hearing loss progression due to over-amplification.

For a child using amplification who experiences a progression in auditory thresholds, the following approach should be taken:

1. Examine middle ear function for negative pressure or fluid.
2. Examine for medical causes of progressive SNHL. Some of these causes include hereditary delayed SNHL, viral infections, hydrops, calcification of the cochlea with meningitis, perilymphatic fistulae, and autoimmune inner ear disease.
3. Remove the hearing aid from the ear with the progression. Have the child continue to wear the other hearing aid and monitor hearing on a weekly basis.

Many times the reason for the progression cannot be ascertained. However, in monitoring over 400 children with SNHL (Pappas ECHO Foundation statistics), progression of the hearing loss reached high proportions in some diagnostic groups (for example, over 50% each in postmeningitic and CMV groups). Not one case has been identified as resulting from powerful hearing aid usage. However, should progression of hearing loss be determined to be related to hearing aid use, it should cause a temporary threshold shift and the hearing thresholds should improve with the removal of the hearing aid

REFERENCES

1. American Academy of Pediatrics Joint Committee on Infant Hearing: Positon Statement, 1994. *Pediatrics.* 1995;95:152-156.
2. American National Standards Institute. Preferred reference quantities for acoustical levels. *ANSI.* New York, American National Standards Institute.1969;8(suppl 1):R 1974.
3. Baloh RW. *Dizziness, Hearing Loss, and Tinnitus: The Essentials of Neurotology.* Philadelphia, Pa: FA Davis; 1984:98.
4. Fria TJ. The assessment of hearing and middle ear function in children. In: Bluestone CD, Stool SE, eds. *Pediatric Otolaryngology.* Philadelphia, Pa: WB Saunders; 1983;1:152-185.
5. Salamy A, Mendelson T, Tooley WH, Choplin E. Contrast in brainstem function between normal and high risk infants in early postnatal life. *Early Hum Dev.* 1980;4:179-185.
6. Mencher GT, Jacobson JT, Seitz MR. Identifying deafness in the newborn. *J Otolaryngol.* 1978;7:490-499.
7. Mencher GT. Perinatal hearing assessment. *Otolaryngol Clin North Am.* 1977;10:177-182.
8. Shulman-Galambos C, Galambos R. Brainstem evoked response audiometry in newborn hearing screening. *Arch Otolaryngol.* 1979;105:86-90.
9. McFarland WH, Simmons FB, Jones FR. An automated hearing screening technique for newborns. *J Speech Hear Disord.* 1980; 45:495-503.

10. Feinmesser M, Tell L. Neonatal screening for detection of deafness. *Arch Oto-laryngol*. 1976;102:297-299.
11. Stewart IF. Newborn infant hearing screening: a five-year pilot project. *J Oto-laryngol*. 1977;6:477-481.
12. Northern JL, Downs MP. *Hearing in Children*. Baltimore, Md: Williams & Wilkins; 1974.
13. Galambos R, Hicks GE, Wilson MJ. Identification audiometry in neonates: a reply to Simmons. *Ear Hear*. 1982;3:189-190.
14. Despland PA, Galambos R. The auditory brainstem response (ABR) is a useful diagnostic tool in the intensive care nursery. *Pediatr Res*. 1980;14:154-158.
15. Pro cit #8.
16. Ling D, Leckie D, Pollack E, et al. Syllable reception by hearing-impaired children trained from infancy in auditory-oral programs. *Volta Rev*. 1981;83:451-457.
17. McConnel F, Liff S. The rationale for early identification and intervention. *Otolaryngol Clin North Am*. 1975;8:77-87.
18. Downs MP. Amplification in the habilitation of the young deaf child. In: Mencher GT, Gerber SE, eds. *Early Management of Hearing Loss*. New York, NY: Grune & Stratton; 1981:199-224.
19. Koenig W. Subjective effects in binaural hearing. *J Acoust Soc Am*. 1950;22: 61-62.
20. Carhart R. Monaural and binaural discrimination against competing sentences. *Int Audiol*. 1965;4:5-10.
21. Pollack I. Monaural and binaural threshold sensitivity for tones and for white noise. *J Acoust Soc Am*. 1948;20:52-57.
22. Reynolds GS, Stevens SS. Binaural summation of loudness. *J Acoust Soc Am*. 1960;32:1334-1337.
23. Markides A. *Binaural Hearing Aids*. New York, NY: Academic Press, 1977.
24. Ross M. A review of studies on the incidence of hearing aid malfunction. *The Condition of Hearing Aids Worn by Children in a Public School Program*. Washington DC: US Government Printing Office; 1977.
25. Gaeth JH, Lounsbury E. Hearing aids and children in elementary schools. *J Speech Hear Disord*. 1966;31:283-289.
26. Zink GK. Hearing aids children wear: a longitudinal study of performance. *Volta Rev*. 1972;74:41-51.
27. Matkin ND. Wearable amplification: a litany of persisting problems. In: Jerger J, ed. *Pediatric Audiology: Current Trends*. San Diego, Ca: College-Hill Press; 1984:125-145.
28. Shephard NT, Gorga MP, Davis JM, Stelmachowicz PG. Characteristics of hearing-impaired children in the public schools. Part 1, Demographic Data. *J Speech Hear Disord*. 1981; 46:123-129.
29. Fletcher SG. Acoustic Phonetics. In: Berg FS, Fletcher SG, eds. *The Hard of Hearing Child*. New York, NY: Grune & Stratton; 1970.
30. Karchmer MA, Kirwin LA. In: *The Use of Hearing Aids by Hearing Impaired Students in the United States*. Washington, DC: Office of Demographic Studies, Gallaudet College; 1977.
31. Ling D, Ling AH. *Aural Habilitation—The Foundations of Verbal Learning in Hearing-Impaired Children*. Washington, DC: Alexander Graham Bell Association for the Deaf; 1978.

32. Op cit #23.
33. Op cit #31.
34. Op cit #31.
35. Kinney CE. Hearing impairments in children. *Laryngoscope*. 1953;63:220-226.
36. Kinney CE. The further destruction of partially deafened children's hearing by the use of powerful hearing aids. *Ann Otol Rhinol Laryngol*. 1961;70: 823-834.
37. Macrae JH, Furrant RH. The effect of hearing aid use on the residual hearing of children with sensorineural deafness. *Ann Otol Rhinol Laryngol*. 1965;74: 409-419.
38. Macrae JH. Deterioration of the residual hearing of children with sensorineural deafness. *Acta Otolaryngol*. 1968;66:33-39.
39. Macrae JH. TTS and recovery from TTS after the use of powerful hearing aids. *J Acoust Soc Am*. 1968;43:145-146.
40. Ross M, Fruex H Jr. Protecting residual hearing in hearing aid users. *Arch Otolaryngol*. 1965;83:165-167.
41. Naunton RF. The effect of hearing aid use upon the user's residual hearing. *Laryngoscope*. 1965;67:165-167.
42. Naunton RF. Deafness in early childhood. In: Lazbi B, ed. *Pediatric Otorhinolaryngology*. New York, NY: Appleton Century Crofts; 1980:13-19.
43. Barr BWE. Prognosis of perceptive hearing loss in children with respect to genesis and use of hearing aid. *Acta Otolaryngol*. 1965;59:462-472.
44. Ross M, Lerman J. Hearing aid usage and its effect on residual hearing: a review of the literature and an investigation. *Arch Otolaryngol*. 1967;86: 639-644.
45. Hawkins DB. Overamplification: a well documented case report. *J Speech Hear Disord*. 1982;47:382-384.

Strategies for Habilitation

Daniel Ling, PhD

Dennis G. Pappas Sr, MD

*What is out of the common is usually a
guide rather than a hindrance.*

A Study in Scarlet
Sherlock Holmes

The habilitation of a child who is hearing-impaired can be carried out in accordance with one of three basic methods: through the use of spoken language, the use of sign language or sign systems, and the simultaneous use of both sign and speech. The basic goal of all three is the development of some form of effective communication. There are very different and strongly conflicting philosophies underlying each of these methods, and the advocates of each method usually accept and promulgate their different philosophies with something approaching religious fervor. This places both the parents of the children and their physicians and audiologists—the first professionals to whom the parents turn for help—in considerable difficulty. Hearing impairment in children is relatively uncommon, so most parents know little or nothing about its implications. Yet it is the parents, not the professionals, who have the responsibility of selecting the type of therapy or education best suited to their children.

CHOOSING A METHOD: A TASK FOR PARENTS

The method parents choose and the outcomes of the type of treatment their children receive will affect their children for the rest of their lives. This being so, professionals must, once a positive diagnosis has been made, ensure that the parents understand the results and ramifications of the diagnostic work they have undertaken, and impartially counsel and advise them on how to best acquire the range of knowledge they must have in order to make informed decisions. None of the methods can meet the individual needs of all children. This being so, our purpose here is to discuss educational methods and their outcomes in relation to the special needs of children with different types and degrees of SNHL.

It would be delightfully simple if each of the three basic types of programs differed only from the others and not within themselves, but that is not the case. There are highly significant variations within each of them. To provide a basic idea of the range of programs available, the names and a brief overview of the different types of programs will be provided here. Later, they will be discussed in detail.

Certain programs focus on the development of spoken language. These include some that concentrate, as far as possible, on the acquisition of auditory skills through the use of hearing aids or cochlear implants. They are called *auditory-verbal* programs. Some so-called *oral* programs focus on the combined use of audition, lipreading (speechreading), and the teaching of speech skills in order to develop spoken language communication. Others use cued speech, an oral system that also employs hand positions and hand configurations as a visual supplement in spoken language communication. Some sign-based programs use only American Sign Language (ASL) for everyday communication, and promote English (which has very different syntax) as a second language through reading and writing, while others use sign systems that employ English syntax and attempt to integrate interpersonal communication skills with the reading and writing of English. The use of sign systems (systems essentially based on ASL, but modified to conform to English grammar) are commonly used in *total communication* programs, which, by definition, are supposed to require the simultaneous use of speech and sign.

The extent to which speech and spoken language communication are encouraged differ greatly from one total communication program to another. In some, the use of speech is strongly encouraged, in others it is neglected. To complicate matters further, the quality of programs of any type are not consistently high.

Before parents make a choice of communication method, they should learn as much as they can about their own child's hearing problems, and the extent to which they can affect the child's reception of spoken language with and without hearing aids. Information beyond that provided by the ear, nose, and throat (ENT) specialist and the audiologist is available from several national organizations. While absorbing such information, they should also learn about and visit the various types of programs available for the treatment of a child such as their own, observe these different sorts of programs in action, talk to parents of children attending them to find out for themselves what skills the children are learning, and how the children interact with each other, their parents, and other adults.

Before a habilitation program has been selected, infants may spend much of their first year communicating without formal language.[1] That is, by using crude signs or speech (reaching and pointing, vocalizations, eye deviations or gaze, facial expressions, gestures, and so forth). The significance of such nonverbal behaviors and the timing of their interaction should not be underrated.[2] The child with hearing impairment may be exceptionally quiet, and parents may have to be encouraged to stimulate nonverbal social interactions with the infant throughout the process of evaluating programs and examining options. Such activity between the infant and parents is often seen at the beginning of auditory training. Undue delays in choosing a communication program may hinder the long-term cognitive development of a child with hearing impairment and should be avoided.

EARLY HABILITATION: A PARENT-INFANT PROGRAM

Children learn language—whether spoken or signed—most readily in the first 2 or 3 years of life. Ideally, therefore, diagnostic assessment and treatment geared toward the development of effective communication skills should begin before a child is more than a few months old (Fig 8–1). Thus, the importance of early habilitation programs serving children with SNHL cannot be overemphasized. Such programs are usually directed toward parents as well as the children, for infants spend most of their time with the family, and it is in the context of everyday family life that they best learn to communicate. Given effective communication, children generally have little or no difficulty acquiring the social and educational skills essential to their development.

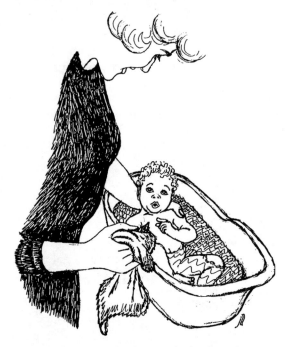

Fig 8-1.—Language development begins through meaningful activity from the earliest stages of infancy.

Early habilitation programs that promote either the use of sign language, spoken language, or both (total communication) are generally available. However, there are many states in which auditory-verbal intervention is not yet available. This we deplore, because the use of modern technology, particularly present-day hearing aids and cochlear implants, makes it possible for the vast majority of children with hearing impairment to acquire a fluent command of spoken language, live first at home, and later follow programs in regular schools. For this reason we shall describe what occurs in a typical auditory-verbal program offering early intervention.

Both the parent and the child, in addition to the educator, are actively involved in the typical 1 or 2 hour weekly auditory-verbal therapy sessions. Techniques to stimulate hearing, speech, and language development are demonstrated by the educator during these sessions and executed and reinforced by the parents during the rest of the week. Children's search for meaning is the driving force for their language acquisition while they are very young. It is not surprising, then, that speech and language are most effectively developed in the context of a child's natural environment. Consequently, parent-infant programs are best carried out in a homelike environment consisting of a model house with typical settings, such as a kitchen, living room, bedroom, and bathroom. When such a facility is not available, therapy sessions should be held in the family's home or a facsimile. Typically, an auditory-verbal program advocates mainstreaming the child who is hearing-impaired into a nursery school for normally hearing children. The purpose of this strategy is to enhance the learning experience of the child who is hearing-impaired by exposing him or her to normally hearing peers. The parent-infant program, with individual therapy, continues in its regular fashion as the child is simultaneously mainstreamed into a regular nursery school.

The importance of daily stimulation by the parents in the process of language acquisition by the very young cannot be overstated. Parent-infant communication is a casual event for the infant with typical hearing; it should be very deliberate in the family of a child who is hearing-impaired. Without a doubt, the parents (or guardians) are the most important participants in the parent-infant program, and their involvement should receive the highest possible priority over children's first 3 years of life. Special demands are placed upon parents and other caregivers for, as their child's natural teachers, it is they who must enhance and reinforce the therapies initiated by the educators. Full-time parent participation in this program is mandatory if maximum remediation of their child's hearing is to be achieved. Early in the parent-infant program, parents learn about hearing and hearing loss. Indeed, many parents become so aware of their child's hearing levels that they are able to detect the slightest indication of progression of the hearing loss, usually reflected in the child's performance.

The ingredients of an effective program are ongoing counseling, continuing educational services, routine and scheduled audiological evaluations, and appropriate otological, psychological, and occupational therapy consultations.

In evaluating the effectiveness of a parent-infant program, the following factors should be considered: the philosophy and goals of the program; the availability of consultants in otology, psychology, and so forth; the procedure or program for audiological reevaluation, including the maintenance and fitting of hearing aids, and tympanometry and audiograms every 6 months; the expertise of the educator in hearing, speech, language, and overall child development; the assessment of progress in speech-language acquisition (preferably every 6 months); and, finally, the evaluation of the speech-language abilities of those students attending the facility, especially those with severe hearing loss.

It must be emphasized that early identification, early amplification, and early training through a parent-infant program is advantageous in all methods of educating those who are hearing-impaired. It is not acceptable to wait or delay these essentials until the child is 3 years old or older. Typically, an auditory program advocates mainstreaming a child with hearing impairment into a nursery school for children who are normally hearing. The purpose of this strategy is to enhance the learning experience of the child who is hearing-impaired by exposing him or her to peers with normal hearing. The infant-parent program, with individual therapy, continues in its regular fashion as the child is simultaneously mainstreamed into a regular nursery school. Children who are hearing-impaired are typically introduced into parent-infant programs as early as 3 months of age.

The central figure in such programs is the auditory-verbal specialist, usually a speech pathologist or specialist teacher of those who are deaf, who undertakes the primary task of counseling the parents and working with the parents and child. It is not unusual for such a program to rely on outside audiologists to select the most appropriate hearing aids or (if the child's hearing impairment is total or near total) service cochlear implants. The more comprehensive auditory-verbal programs, however, coordinate or offer a wide range of services, including those of pediatric audiologists, educators, speech pathologists, and even, in some cases, otologists, psychologists, and occupational therapists. In these programs, the parents are seen as the primary agents of habilitation, as they are with the children most of their waking hours. They learn how to verify that the child's hearing aids or cochlear implants work well, how to use them to optimum advantage in developing communication skills in the course of interactions within the home and family, how to take care of these instruments, and how to carry out ongoing evaluation of their child's progress. Usually, early auditory-verbal programs accept children from the first few months of age and continue to monitor the progress of the children and offer the family support services after the child enters school. Most children who attend such programs throughout their early years enter regular schools. An important part of the program's work, therefore, is to establish a liaison with these local schools so that well-informed regular teachers are available to the children once they reach school age.

EDUCATIONAL PLACEMENT OF SCHOOL-AGED CHILDREN

The government has played a vital part in the improvement of educational placements for children who are hearing-impaired. In accordance with the mandate of Public Law 94-142, special educational programming must be available to them in the least restrictive environment, and parents, as well as professionals, are expected to contribute to the design of each child's individual education plan (IEP). The team preparing the plan may include a variety of specialists, including a special educator for those who are hearing-impaired. If appropriate, the child must be given the opportunity of being educated with their normally hearing peers. The student with hearing impairment who requires the academic support of a special educator may be placed in a self-contained classroom and integrated with the students who are normally hearing in nonacademic classes such as art and physical education.

The opportunity afforded by this mandate takes effect when a child who is hearing-impaired reaches grade school. Prior to that time (from birth to 6 years) there is no mandate for mainstreaming and programs are built not so much around a method, but around the philosophies and skills of the professional providing the leadership—in some cases a physician and in others the speech-language pathologist or a specialist teacher of those who are deaf who provides the therapy. Implementation of a mainstreaming program varies according to the educational philosophies of the person providing leadership. It is usually stressed by auditory-verbal therapists, most of whom work on a one-to-one basis and can be expected to be certified by Auditory-Verbal International, the organization that sets the accepted standards for such work. Although some multisensory (oral) and total communication programs advocate individualized treatment on a one-to-one basis in a parent-infant program, others encourage a classroom setting of groups of children who are hearing-impaired. Primary placements in nursery schools may include a special class for those who are hearing-impaired, rather than a setting for youngsters with normal hearing.

The goal of mainstreaming is to promote the fullest development of the potential of a child who is hearing-impaired. For some this goal is met by full-time integration with students who are normally hearing; for others, a program of partial integration would be more appropriate.[3]

Awareness of the extensive range of individual needs among children has been widespread for many years. It is a tradition in our society that parents, in seeking to meet the needs of their children in an optimal manner, should have the right to choose among different types of programs and to express not only their preferences for a particular type of program, but for that program to cater to their child's individual differences and needs. This right is embodied in Public Law 94-142 and, as mentioned, such choices are reflected in the basic requirements for structuring IEPs. Among the many papers on the topic of educational placement, one written a quarter of a century ago by Deno substantially influenced thinking about the various types of programs required to accommodate the widely different needs of children with all types of disability. Deno[4] proposed a cascade model of provision, one that recognized all levels of provision as essential, but regular school placement as the most desirable and other placements as less desirable forms of provision. The model, translated into modern terms, looked like this:

▶ Regular class in regular school with no support services
▶ Regular classes in regular schools with essential support services
▶ Special class in regular school with children mainstreamed for certain lessons
▶ Day schools for children with special needs
▶ Residential special schools
▶ Hospital or home-based special education
▶ Custodial care

Mainstreaming and Other Strategies

Of course, mainstreamed settings are the least restrictive educational environment for children who are able to cope without undue difficulty in regular schools and classes. If there are difficulties, mainstreamed settings can still provide the least restrictive environment for children provided support services (audiology, speech pathology, access to special teaching, and so on) are made available to them. Mainstreaming children who are hearing-impaired can be undertaken in a variety of ways, regardless of the communication method employed. Children attending regular schools without school-based support services have to be able to communicate through speech. Children who use other methods of communication (sign or cued speech) require translators or transliterators as part of their support services. Teachers who have children with hearing impairment in their regular classes should be well-acquainted with their special needs. In short, they should:

▶ Be aware of the facts and implications of hearing impairment in childhood;
▶ Understand the fundamentals of classroom acoustics; be familiar with a child's amplification systems (personal aids and FM device and radio microphone), know how to check that the amplification systems are in good working order, and how to use them to optimal advantage;
▶ Be positive about having a child who is hearing-impaired in the class; know that teacher attitudes toward such children will be reflected in other students' behaviors;
▶ Expect the same standards of academic and personal behavior from children who are hearing-impaired as from others in the class; and
▶ Expect children who are hearing-impaired to participate fully in and beyond the classroom.

The special class in a regular school has many advantages. It permits the employment of a specialist teacher who is always on-site and available to both teachers and pupils. It also permits increase in mainstream activities as the child develops the required coping skills, first in classes such as physical education, art, and games in which communication is least important, and later in some, or all, academic subjects. Parent guidance can be provided at each successive stage of a child's development. In addition to input from their teachers, children with hearing impairment attending regular classes on a full- or part-time basis can benefit from some sort of buddy system. In addition to formal support services, it is most helpful if other children in the regular class are also available to:

▶ Explain the class rules;
▶ Ensure that announcements are understood;
▶ Make carbons or photocopies of notes;
▶ Ensure that the child who is hearing-impaired knows about all the school's student services;
▶ Make sure that out-of-school functions are brought to the attention of the child with hearing impairment;
▶ Act as occasional tutors; and
▶ Help if directions are missed or misunderstood.

Full-time placements in special classes or special schools (day or residential) do not demand that a particular type of communication be used. Exemplary schools that use auditory-verbal, oral, cued speech, and sign are to be found in various locations across North America. The communication system habitually used by peers is, however, a very strong influence on the type of communication system the child will develop and prefer. Thus, self-contained schools and classes in which children are not constantly surrounded and engaged in speech communication involving normally hearing adults and peers are not the easiest environments in which to stimulate spoken language development. For this reason it is unusual, but not impossible, to find residential schools for children with hearing impairment in which spoken language is the primary means of communication both during and outside school hours. Children with profound hearing loss who talk may even lose their spoken language skills when placed in residential school environments in which sign language is used in class and predominates in the residences. Hospital and home-based education, as well as custodial care for individual school-aged children who are hearing-impaired, can also feature any desired form of communication. Home-based education is not uncommon, and, in fact, is highly recommended for infants and children under school age when such treatment is part of a well-organized parent-child intervention program.

The opportunities afforded by Public Law 94-142 take effect when children are old enough to enter grade school. Prior to that time (from birth to 6 years) there is no mandate for educational placement in the least restrictive environment (LRE). Implementation of a mainstreaming program by individual systems varies according to educational philosophies. Typically, an auditory-verbal program advocates mainstreaming the child who is hearing-impaired into a nursery school for children with normal hearing. The purpose of this strategy is to enhance the learning experience of the child who is hearing-impaired by exposing him or her to peers who are normally hearing. Most parent-infant programs that feature auditory-verbal therapy continue individual therapy when the child is simultaneously mainstreamed into a regular nursery school. Some multisensory (oral) and total communication programs run their own individually based parent-infant programs, while others encourage group instruction of children who are hearing-impaired. For some, full-time integration with normally hearing students is appropriate; for others, a program of partial integration is more efficient.

As noted, the concept of *inclusion* is by no means new. It was certainly envisaged by Deno in the first two (or even three) categories of her Cascade Model. The idea of teaching children with and without special needs together in regular school classes goes back well beyond the beginning of this century. It derives essentially from the notion that schools should reflect the structure of (represent the proportion of sensorily or physically challenged individuals in) society at large. The inclusion movement in the United States was stimulated in the 1980s by then Assistant Secretary for Special Education, Madeline Wills, who advocated full mainstreaming of children with disabilities, a movement that became known as the regular education initiative (REF). The idea is not to ignore individual differences and needs, but to have all teachers and children recognize and respect them, and to have them met in a regular school environment with all children participating in both in-school and extracurricular activities. For the REF to be effective, regular and special educational practices have to complement each other; appropriate individualized instruction must be formulated and provided through the IEP process; and regular class teachers, parents, and the children with special needs must receive the support services they require. This is a tall order, particularly for helping children with severe or profound hearing impairment, who constitute about 0.01% of the population, when there is a shortage of funding and an even greater shortage of specially trained personnel to provide the necessary support services. Accordingly, there are severe risks of children with special needs being inappropriately placed in restrictive learning environments and even sacrificing the educational standards of their normal peers. It is not unheard of for some school boards to use the REF as a means to save funds by cutting special educational services and ignoring special needs.

In order for mainstreaming to be effective, attention has to be paid to several factors regardless of the communication mode employed. These include the:

▶ Level of the child's academic knowledge and personal-social skills;
▶ Extent and quality of family participation;
▶ Physical environment (structure, acoustic treatment, and lighting of the classroom, distances and distractions);
▶ Teacher's qualities, including skills, style and attitudes;
▶ Organization of instruction (number of classes, individual study conditions);
▶ Administrative aspects (knowledge, understanding, experience, and willingness of administrators and boards);
▶ Support services available (audiological, social, occupational and other therapies.); and
▶ Miscellaneous details, such as transport, special clothing, and costs.

Educational Methods Based on Speech and Spoken Language

Speech and language are terms that are often confused or used interchangeably. Language is a mentally based phenomenon consisting of words and the rules governing their use. Speech is simply one physical way of expressing language. Language can also be expressed in writing or in sign. Languages differ primarily from one country to another, but most of the speech sounds used to express the various different languages are similar, if not identical. Reading and writing are usually developed through reference to the spoken language children have learned at an earlier stage of development. We use the term spoken language throughout this chapter to avoid confusion with the expression of language through either speech or sign.

The levels of language skills required for adequate speech communication are relative rather than absolute.[5] For instance, in the child with normal hearing, first words may be intelligible only to the mother and no one else. Normally hearing children, in their early years, understand and are understood through the confines of their limited vocabulary and grammar. Attempts to study the language-learning process in children who are normal hearing led to the development of a discipline known as psycholinguistics. Noam Chomsky, a pioneer in this field, directed his investigations toward understanding the manner in which language is acquired, rather than studying the actual utterances that emerge in its use. Today, language development is also studied in terms of pragmatic teaching procedures aimed at refining linguistic skills. The study of psycholinguistics, then, has provided the much needed impetus for the study of language skills of children with hearing impairment.

Several successful approaches to teaching speech and spoken language have been designed. Those of Ling, Pollack, and Beebe have been adopted internationally. Using speech in the acquisition of language has been stressed by Ling,[6] whose system for teaching speech skills is systematically related to the semantic, pragmatic, and syntactic aspects of language. Ling's program[7] has been widely adopted by educators using auditory-verbal, traditional oral, and total communication modes of instruction. In implementing such a program, sequential 6-month evaluations of progress in cognitive development must be monitored. According to Ling and Milne,[5] problems in the spoken language of children who are hearing-impaired become evident when the following five conditions exist:

▶ When their vocabulary is limited for their age group;
▶ When their expressions consist, either in whole or in part, of immature or abnormal syntactic structures;
▶ When their pragmatic use of language is deviant;
▶ When they cannot realize their semantic intentions because their cognition (thought) far outstrips their word knowledge and linguistic skills, and
▶ When phonology does not approximate the adult form as closely as that of their hearing peers.

Judgment of whether meaningful speech and language exists must be made relative to the child's age (Fig 8–2). Because of the dependence on speech communication in day-to-day life, the development of intelligible speech is important for all children and critical for children with hearing impairment. It is a goal to be sought vigorously in every type of program.

Speech is part of the curriculum of most educational programs for those who are hearing-impaired. Regardless of educational philosophies, most professionals working with children who are hearing-impaired recognize that those who can communicate through the use of spoken language have many advantages. They can interact more freely with other members of society, most of whom talk. They can, therefore, function more independently in most of the circumstances that they are likely to meet in life. Legislation and social awareness have improved the lot of

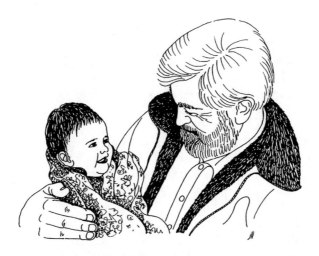

Fig 8-2.—Daniel Ling developing early use of spoken language with a child who is hearing-impaired.

most people who are hearing-impaired in Western societies but, even so, the advantages lie with those who can talk. With spoken language, opportunities for higher education are less restricted, a more extensive range of careers is open, and there is greater security of employment. Those who can talk also face fewer limitations in the personal and social aspects of their lives.[8]

Methods of teaching spoken language to children with impaired hearing, the so-called oral methods, have been known and applied since the 17th century.[9] Such work originally focused mainly on visual means of teaching, the written form and lipreading (speechreading), though tactile cues were also employed as a means of perceiving and producing speech. The task of teaching through the use of vision and touch is a slow one and it is virtually impossible for children with little or no hearing to learn language spontaneously by such means. Teachers therefore tended to approach their teaching task analytically: to develop language through reference to grammatical rules and to develop speech one sound at a time, combining each sound into words as soon as possible. This approach became known as the structural (or analytical) method. In contrast, some teachers advocated a natural (or synthetic) method, one in which language was taught through the process of communication and speech through the correction of the child's attempts to use words. The natural method was first mentioned by Delgarno in 1680 and later practiced by Alexander Graham Bell.[10]

Although Alexander Graham Bell is most widely remembered for inventing the telephone, he also became famous for teaching children who were hearing-impaired to talk. He was an exceptionally confident speech teacher. In his book, *The Mechanism of Speech*, he does not question the notion that "deaf" children can learn to talk intelligibly. He even cautions that, when working with children who were hearing-impaired, one should seek to obtain from them "not the speech of the elocutionist, but the speech of the people among whom the children live." [10,p14]

During the past century, research has led to greatly increased knowledge relating to linguistics. It has also led to numerous technological developments. As a result, we are now in a much better position than Bell and, indeed than workers at any other time in history, to promote the development of speech communication skills among children who are hearing-impaired. As compared with Bell, we know much more about the acquisition of spoken language; we now have devices that can be used to measure hearing, amplify speech for the listener with hearing impairment, use electrical currents to stimulate receptors in the inner ear through cochlear implants, and transmit speech to the skin through vibrotactile or electrotactile stimulation. Such products of technology, many of them originating in Bell's work, provide enormous opportunities for teachers, clinicians, and parents as they struggle to find increasingly effective ways to promote spoken language.

Auditory-Verbal (Unisensory, Acoupedic) Programs

Auditory-verbal programs are the most recently developed form of educational treatment for children who are hearing-impaired. As the term *auditory-verbal* suggests, these programs focus to the greatest extent possible on the use of children's residual hearing and the development of their spoken language skills. To achieve such focus, professionals in auditory-verbal therapy/teaching suppress the use of vision (speechreading) during training periods, both as part of ongoing diagnosis and as a training procedure that helps children to use their residual hearing and understand speech. Such an approach has become feasible only over the past few decades. It was not until well into the 20th century that technological devices such as the audiometer and hearing aids were developed, and it became possible to measure and use children's residual hearing. It is only in recent years that computer technology has permitted the measurement of newborn infants' hearing through use of ABR testing, evaluation of hearing through OAEs, the use of probe-tube microphones for the objective measurement of sound pressures in the ear canal, new types of hearing aids, and the development of cochlear implants.

Auditory-verbal programs are appropriate for two types of children: those who have sufficient useful residual hearing to permit them, when adequately aided, to hear most of the patterns of speech; and those who, though totally or near-totally deaf, are fitted with cochlear implants, and are thus similarly able to perceive the patterns of spoken language. With today's hearing aids and cochlear implants, this covers the majority of children with hearing impairment. Auditory-verbal programs developed essentially as an outcome of the effort of creative teachers and clinicians to make the most effective use of available technology as a means of helping children who are hearing-impaired become well-adjusted, fully integrated, communicating and contributing members of our hearing society. This approach now enables the majority of children who are hearing-impaired, from an early age to perceive and produce normal or near-normal spoken language and to acquire higher levels of speech communication skills with less difficulty than ever before. What was highly appropriate in the treatment of children with hearing impairment some few years ago may no longer be so. Emerging technology is and will continue to be constantly driving clinical and educational practices toward fundamental change and improvement. Never in the history of education of the deaf have there been greater opportunities and potential for the optimal personal, social, and educational development for children with hearing impairment.

The application of modern technology favors spoken language communication through auditory-verbal development over all other alternatives for children who are hearing-impaired, essentially because the technologies in our field are concerned with processing signals that are acoustic rather than visual. The effective use of technology together with early intervention provides highly advantageous conditions for auditory-verbal development, mainly because children learn language most readily in the first few years of life, and because it is during infancy that mothers and children are constantly in close contact—a condition that provides the best possible acoustic conditions for speech perception.

The early development of language and communication can minimize later educational problems, for only if there is effective communication can there be optimal learning. Most babies who are hearing-impaired fitted with appropriate hearing aids in early infancy are enabled not only to hear the speech of others around them, but to monitor the sounds they inadvertently make or deliberately babble and associate the sounds with spoken language and sound that relates to objects, events, and people around them. In order for early treatment to be effective, one of the professionals' primary concerns must be with helping parents understand how best to help their child develop communication skills as part of their overall development. Auditory-verbal programs are based on the following principles:

▶ Early identification of hearing impairment through screening tests of hearing in newborn and other infants.
▶ Early and aggressive medical and audiological management.
▶ Selection and adjustment of appropriate hearing aids or, if necessary, cochlear implants to ensure that children optimally hear their own and others' spoken language.
▶ Making sound, particularly the sounds of spoken language, meaningful. Ensuring optimal development of speech and spoken language and personal-social skills.
▶ Providing counseling and support services to enable parents to serve as the primary agents in children's habilitation.
▶ Pursuing programs of ongoing diagnosis in the course of treatment.
▶ Supplying support services for children so that they can participate educationally and socially with children attending typical (regular) education classes.

To be exquisitely successful, auditory-verbal treatment must begin in early infancy when children are most receptive to learning spoken language. Thus, physicians can make a substantial contribution to their success through willingness to establish programs of early identification and diagnosis. The current trend in the United States of America and in Canada is toward the testing of all infants using physiological indicators such as ABR and OAEs. There are now automatic ABR screening instruments that can be effectively used by intelligent volunteers with relatively little training. Such instruments can, in about 3–4 minutes per infant, provide an objective and highly reliable pass/fail decision on most children tested during the first few days of life. OAEs are generated by the hair cells in the cochlea when they are stimulated by sound. Instruments that present sounds to a listener by sweeping pure tones at all frequencies across the speech spectrum and automatically recording the responses of the hair cells can be used to test cochlear integrity. These are the measures that are recommended by the US National Institutes of Health (NIH) consensus development conference on early identification of hearing impairment in infants and young children. Free single copies of the *NIH Consensus Statement on the Early Identification of Hearing Impairment in Infants and Young Children* (1994) can be obtained from the office of Medical Applications of Research, NIH, Federal Building, Room 618, Bethesda, MD, 20892, USA, (301) 496-1143.

Although auditory-verbal work holds more promise of successful habilitation than previously designed programs, it must be recognized that no one method or collection of methods can possibly meet the educational needs of all children with impaired hearing, because the extent of disability and the range of additional problems associated or not with the hearing loss is quite large. Not all children, therefore, meet the necessary conditions for successful auditory-verbal work, such as early identification and diagnosis, sufficient useful residual hearing when appropriately aided or the use of cochlear implants, and parents who seek that form of treatment and choose to become the primary caregivers and agents of habilitation. For such children, alternative means of acquiring spoken language that feature more traditional methods of therapy and education are available. These are discussed below.

Traditional Oral Methods

Over the course of its long history, traditional oral methods have, at one time or another, incorporated the use of all sensory modalities (Fig 8–3).

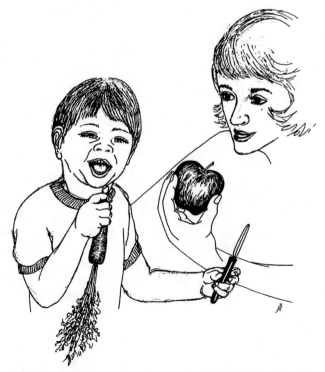

Fig 8-3.—Parents are the primary agents in developing their children's spoken language through ongoing stimulation in meaningful situations.

When different emphases have been placed on certain sensory modalities, oral programs have been said to use oral-ocular, oral-aural (oral auditory), lipreading (speechreading) and multisensory methods.

Until relatively recently, oral education was provided mainly in special schools and classes catering to children from kindergarten through to the upper grades. When pupils were ready to leave school, they would go on to either further education or to work. Very similar, somewhat formal, methods of teaching were adhered to throughout the school lives of the children enrolled. Some such schools still exist.

Traditional oral methods tended to include more emphasis on lipreading than the use of hearing and to focus more strongly than auditory-verbal programs on the written form as an important aid to language learning. This is, of course, to be expected, because such methods were designed over a hundred years before technologies that allowed the use of residual hearing became available. Traditional oral schools consistently had as their purpose the preparation of their students for life in society at large. Their goals were to produce children with a good knowledge of language, intelligible speech, and sufficient education to have a successful career and enjoy a happy personal life. However, they did not usually have the luxury of selecting their students, so these goals were not always achieved by those who were not gifted. Inevitably, some such pupils failed to acquire good spoken language skills and an adequate education. On the other hand, a fair proportion of graduates from traditional oral schools also went on to professional occupations such as medicine, dentistry, chemistry, law, education, and agricultural science. Hundreds of such professionals are members of the Oral Deaf Adults Society of the Alexander Graham Bell Association for the Deaf.

For well over a century oral schools tended to be somewhat isolated institutions—backwaters in which their teachers felt little or no obligation to attend to mainstream educational thought. This is no longer so. Although modern and tradition oral programs have much in common, the current thrust of technological progress, the outcomes of early auditory-verbal intervention, and the drive towards mainstreaming has been recognized and welcomed by progressive oral programs. Many of them admit children who have received early auditory-verbal therapy but are not yet ready for enrollment in mainstream education, and most admit children well before they reach kindergarten age—indeed, as soon as they are diagnosed. Many such children have too little hearing or have some other form of handicap that renders them unable to benefit adequately from auditory-verbal treatment. They have to be taught through more traditional oral methods that include greater focus on vision and touch if they are to acquire speech communication skills and satisfactory levels of education. Present day oral programs for such children focus on lipreading while using hearing aids as a supplement in speech perception and develop speech and language through more formal work. Since few children have total hearing loss in the low frequency range, the voice quality of children in any type of program will reflect the amount of auditory experience the program is able to provide.

Speech perception and speech production, plus the comprehension of language, are basic concerns in oral programs. Speech is processed at several levels: *detection* (can the speech pattern be detected through audition, vision, or touch?); *discrimination* (can one speech pattern be differentiated from another through one or more of the sensory modalities?); *identification* (can particular sounds be recognized for what they are?); and *comprehension* (are the speech patterns presented to the child meaningful and understood?). In treating children who are hearing-impaired, one should attend mainly to detection and comprehension. With detection, one should ensure that, through the use of the most appropriate sensory aids, the fullest possible range of sounds is available to the child and that the child is encouraged to actively use the senses (listening, looking, and feeling, rather than hearing, seeing, and touching). Attention in everyday life can then be given to the most important and highest level of processing, that of comprehension, which involves the analysis of running speech (not isolated sounds), as well as cognitive (problem-solving and conceptual) activity and linguistic (pragmatic, semantic, syntactic, and phonological) skills and their development.

Speechreading (Lipreading)

Lipreading is essential for spoken language communication when residual hearing is inadequate for the comprehension of speech. However, it has serious weaknesses because many speech patterns that sound different (eg, /p/, /b/, /m/ and /t/, /s/, /d/, /n/) look alike on the lips. Even so, most people use speechreading under certain circumstances. Of the seven aspects of speech described above, vocalization and voice patterns (intonation, duration, intensity, and stress) cannot be seen, vowels are but partly discernible through vision (tongue position, which is crucial, is often masked by the lips and teeth), and only place of consonant production is relatively visible. Speechreading can successfully function as the major input modality only when:

▶ Hearing aids are used to amplify an existing fragments of audition;
▶ Linguistic cues are available;
▶ Topical knowledge is provided;

▶ Situational background and ongoing activities provide context; and
▶ Prevailing social and educational subjects are the focus of the conversation.

Many oral programs use visual aids in addition to lipreading. As each visual aid has been devised, difficulties have been experienced in its use. The most serious difficulty with visual aids, including currently available computerized aids that provide visual images of different speech patterns, relate to the inherent complexity and integrity of the speech signal. The more complete the speech pattern displayed, the more difficult it is for children to use it to their advantage; and the simpler the pattern displayed, the less adequately it represents everyday speech. Most visual aids have been designed for speech training rather than as instruments for use in everyday situations. It is difficult to promote the carryover of speech skills into everyday life when they are learned through strategies that do not involve interpersonal communication (Fig 8–4).[11]

Oral-Tactile-Kinesthetic Procedures

When we talk, we create speech patterns that cannot only be heard and seen, but speech patterns that can also be felt. Just as every speech pattern sounds different to the normal listener, so it feels different to the speaker.

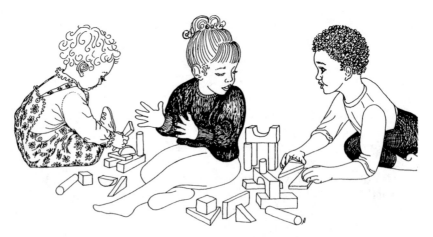

Fig 8-4.—Interaction with hearing peers promotes the carryover of speech skills into everyday life. Many modern oral schools program both educational and social integration opportunities for their children with hearing impairment.

Those of us who have normal hearing are not very aware of how our speech feels when we talk. We attend more to how it sounds. But, unconsciously, we are very "tuned in" to the way our speech organs touch each other (create tactile sensations) and move (create kinesthetic sensations) as we speak. This is clearly shown by those who are unfortunate enough to lose all of their hearing as adults. They do not stop talking. Nor does their speech become unintelligible. They continue to talk, and can do so because they are guided by the tactile and kinesthetic sensations they have long been accustomed to perceiving, perhaps without knowing it. In contrast, children who lose their hearing when they are too young to have had extensive experience of tactile and kinesthetic sensations may, in the absence of appropriate help, also lose their speech because they have no proprioception to guide them when audition has been lost.[8]

One of the most important aspects of work on speech development with children who are hearing-impaired is to establish articulatory coding: a repertoire of tactile and kinesthetic sensations that can, even in the complete absence of hearing, serve as a reliable guide for speech production. If appropriate training promotes awareness of the way correct speech patterns feel, children who become totally deaf following meningitis or some other disease, as well as those who have been profoundly hearing-impaired from birth, can learn how to produce intelligible speech through self-monitoring. At first, this may require the sensations created by speaking to be the focus of their conscious attention. Later, when speech becomes an automatic act, attention is more usually concentrated on what one is saying than on determining its long-term effects on speech production.[12]

Touch can be used in developing the speech reception and speech production of youngsters who have hearing impairment. Children can be encouraged to consciously feel what certain speech patterns are like when others produce them. Voicing can be felt on the chest, pitch can be felt as an elevation of the larynx, the tongue's position for various vowels can be felt with a finger in the mouth when the lips and teeth do not permit it to be seen, the burst of air can be detected when plosives such as /p/ and /t/ are sounded out, and the flow of air can be felt on a wet fingertip when fricatives like /s/ and /f/ are produced. Natural touch can also provide the child with an analog of a sound's duration or intensity as a finger is drawn slowly or quickly, lightly or heavily, down the arm or across the palm of a child's hand. Speech rhythms can be similarly indicated by tapping the pattern on the child's wrist or knee. More formalized ways of using touch (eg, the Tadoma method) have long been used to convey speech to those who neither hear nor see.

Time-honored tactile strategies of the type described above remain necessary for some children. The more profoundly hearing-impaired the child, the more likely it is that, in spite of technological advances, some use of human touch will be helpful in his or her development of speech. Because such strategies are old, they are not necessarily out of date.[11]

Tactile devices have emerged as wearable instruments only during the past few years. Traditionally, touch was a close sense that demanded direct contact. Technology has essentially changed this, and allows touch to function, along with hearing and sight, as a third distance sense. A microphone can be made to feed an amplifier which, in turn, can be made to feed receivers of some sort that will vibrate the skin, or energize electrodes that will cause a small electric current to flow onto the skin. The quite distant acoustic events that surround us can thus be brought to the body and represented as a series of tactile stimuli. Some form of coding is essential if speech is to be transmitted via the skin, because the skin is incapable of receiving and permitting discrimination of the intensity, duration and, particularly, frequency components of speech in their raw form.[13] Tactile devices therefore tend to use place of contact on the skin to represent the frequency (spectral) components of speech. Some workers have demonstrated that there are many similarities between tactile and auditory speech reception, and wearable tactile devices have shown promise as supplements to speechreading.[14] Many types of wearable tactile devices are now in use, and those with several channels (vibrators or electrodes) can be used in everyday communicative experience as well as through formal teaching.[11]

Cued Speech

The system known as *cued speech* was introduced by Cornett in 1967.[15] Its purpose is to eliminate the ambiguity in speechreading by providing a variety of hand cues simultaneously with the spoken message. Just as letters and numbers can be used together to create a grid that specifies the exact location of a place on a map, lipreading and the hand cues provided by cued speech can specify exactly which vowels, diphthongs, and consonants are being produced by a talker. Shapes that look alike on the lips are associated with different hand positions or configurations. The hand cues are not signs; they have no intrinsic meaning in and of themselves. They are made only to resolve the confusions existing among the speech segments as they appear in lipreading.

Cued speech can permit the reception of speech by school-aged children with no or totally or nearly no hearing at extremely high (greater than 90%) levels of accuracy.[16] Some professionals have reported that the system tends to encourage children to become so visual that they do not attend adequately to the acoustic aspects of speech, such as prosody, that are best perceived through the use of residual hearing. Indeed, vocalization and prosody cannot be cued effectively, and hence the voice quality of children taught by this means may be poor. Further research is required to determine whether cued speech creates such disadvantages among children who have useful residual hearing, or use cochlear implants or tactile aids, and to determine its long-term effects on speech production.[8]

Traditional Manual Methods

Sign Language(Manual Language and Fingerspelling)

Gesture has been a part of human communication throughout recorded history. There is no account of when it was first used in the process of teaching children with impaired hearing. The first educator known to state a preference for the use of manual language for the purpose of teaching such children was Juan Pablo Bonet, a Spaniard, who wrote a book on his method in 1620.[17] Bonet used a multisensory method with his pupils: He read letters and words aloud to them while using the finger configurations on one hand to spell the letters of the alphabet, while pointing to the letters and words he was attempting to teach with the other hand. Thus fingerspelling was the first manual method. Communicating by spelling out a message one letter at a time is a very slow process but, nevertheless, its use along with speech was later adopted in North America and persisted well into this century. Speech with fingerspelling is known as the Rochester method. The use of this method is not currently widespread. Nowadays, fingerspelling is more commonly used along with sign language to specify particular words for which there is no sign or to avoid or resolve ambiguity when signing.

Sign language, the use of physical gestures to specify particular words, became widespread following its adoption as a teaching tool by the Abbé de L'Epée, who founded a public school for deaf children in Paris, in 1755. His purpose was fundamentally a religious one—by teaching persons with hearing impairment to communicate and thus to be able to take their vows, he could save their souls. Prior to this time, the fate of the souls of the deaf were considered to be somewhat in question. The Abbé de L'Epée did not use signs to the exclusion of speech as some advocate today and, in fact, wrote very insightfully on techniques for developing speech skills. Sign language was introduced in the United States in 1817, in the American Asylum for the Deaf and Dumb when it was founded by Thomas Hopkins Gallaudet in Hartford, Connecticut, in 1817.[18] The use of sign language in schools and colleges segregated from society at-large led, in general, to the decline of speech communication skills and to the creation of a group of people who were unable to communicate with people having typical hearing. Thus, a secondary result of segregated schools and colleges solely for those who are deaf (recently Gallaudet College in Washington, DC was awarded university status) was to create and perpetuate a subculture of persons who were deaf and who looked to others who were educated as themselves for mutual support and a congenial context for personal-social growth. Those who identify themselves with this subculture prefer to call themselves Deaf (with a capital D) rather than hearing-impaired, even though surveys carried out by Gallaudet University show that many individuals who are Deaf have less severe hearing loss than people who have been treated in auditory-verbal or other oral programs and are elsewhere considered to have hearing impairment rather than Deafness.

The sign language used in schools and colleges that were segregated from society inevitably led to the growth of a specifically American form of sign language. American Sign Language (Ameslan or ASL), sometimes augmented by fingerspelling, has become a viable, self-contained language in its own right. Pride in their subculture and in their language has recently led many people who are Deaf to completely reject the development of speech skills and to advocate a form of bilingualism, one in which everyday communication is carried out in ASL and reading and writing are carried out in English. Since the two languages are distinct in their grammar and syntax (ASL does not have the same word order as English, omitting articles and certain verb tenses), this places a particularly heavy burden on children whose academic education must inevitably wait on the acquisition of a written form of a foreign language. The outcome of this development has yet to be studied.[19]

Total Communication (Combined or Simultaneous Method)

Manual communication (sign language and fingerspelling), speechreading, and auditory training through amplification are all employed in the total communication method for educating children with hearing impairment. One of the main drives toward the widespread adoption of total communication in North America was the appallingly low educational standards that prevailed in schools—particularly state schools for the deaf. Many such schools were designated as oral schools, and hence were considered to be producing oral failures. But in fact most of the children in these schools were using ASL, a language incompatible with spoken English. To make sign compatible with spoken English and thus facilitate the simultaneous presentation of the two forms of communication, several sign systems were developed, notably SEE-1 and SEE-2.[20] Proponents of total communication claim that the use of a sign system (as compared with a sign language) in combination with speech will enhance the meaningfulness of residual hearing and lipreading. However, about half of the children in total communication programs do not develop intelligible speech. Such children may read, write, and sign without meaningfully using the spoken word.[21]

It is difficult to present sign and speech together. Even the most fluent signers tend to speak in an abnormal manner when using any sign system. Several different systems have therefore been designed and applied. Among them are *Seeing Essential English* (SEE-1). SEE-1 is used as a supplement to speech and language and speechreading in many schools and clinics. It incorporates English word parts such as prefixes, roots, or suffixes, and verb tenses, which are indicated by a sign to indicate appropriate grammatical endings (that is, -ed or -ing).[22] *Signing Exact English* (SEE-2) is signed as it is spoken. Signs in this system are designed to translate English in such a way that word order and word equivalence, rather than just the roots of words, are presented, as in SEE-1. SEE-2, which is said to be easy for parents to learn, attempts to remain as close as possible to traditional signing while following its own principles.[23] Both forms of SEE signing are faster methods than fingerspelling and are easier to read. However, they are not as fast as ASL.

In addition to the sign systems and fingerspelling mentioned above, Pidgin Sign English (PSE), has also been developed. It has progressed from being a jargon form of signing to its current usage as a combination of attempts to employ the English grammatical structure with SEE-2 while maintaining the conceptual base of ASL.

Research from various sources, including Gallaudet University, has shown that total communication has not improved the overall poor academic achievement of students who are deaf and have left school across the country and has left many children with hearing impairment with very low-level communication skills. Many parents, particularly those of children attending residential special schools, have not learned to communicate with sign language sufficiently to maintain a close relationship with their children during their school years. Comparison of academic and communicative performance of children taught through total communication and in up-to-date oral programs strongly favor the latter. Placement in special schools for students who are deaf is a very costly way for states to provide substandard education for many children with hearing impairment. Costs often exceed $50000 per pupil. The strongest argument for the continuation of total communication as the only or primary option in many states seems to be that it is administratively convenient for school boards. Many of them apparently like to offer just the one monolithic system that claims to provide (though it cannot) appropriate education for all children by giving emphasis to whatever aspects of the method most readily meets the needs of a particular child, regardless of the degree of hearing impairment or the extent of additional disabilities. It is not surprising that in recent years total communication has received an increasing amount of criticism both from the community of those who are Deaf[24] and from scientists who hear.[19]

Speech competence does not necessarily depend on the degree of hearing impairment.[25] Factors that influence speech and spoken language development include the possible presence of additional disabilities, the instructional language program used, the competence of the educator, and the extent of parental involvement. Such "variant problems" may impede the development of a child who is hearing-impaired, regardless of the type of program selected. Although they are extremely demanding on resources, the auditory-verbal and oral tradition of early education for those who are hearing-impaired are not necessarily more expensive than the cost of placing somewhat older children in residential special schools and training students with hearing impairment to become lifelong members of a subculture such as for individuals who are Deaf.

The arguments for and against auditory-verbal and traditional oral programs relative to total communication programs are far-reaching. Many of them make little sense because children's futures should not be shaped according to the nature of available prefabricated programs, but according to the children's demonstrated individual needs. Only two basic principles need to be generally agreed upon:

▶ Children who are hearing-impaired who have the potential ability to learn to speak and to understand speech should be given the opportunity to do so,[12] and

▶ Greatest emphasis on the acquisition of speech is found in auditory-verbal and modern oral programs.

PSYCHOLOGY OF CHILDREN WITH HEARING IMPAIRMENT

Psychological Ramifications of SNHL: Signs and Symptoms

The population of children with SNHL is characterized by a vast range of individual differences and individual needs. The type and degree of hearing impairment may vary from one child to another, and such variation alone results in individual differences of sufficient proportions to justify a wide range of educational programming. However, hearing loss, itself, may cause secondary intellectual, learning, or social problems. Further, hearing impairment and other additional physical, sensory, and/or intellectual problems may share a common cause. For this latter reason, neurological examination of children with SNHL is recommended, for neurological deficits may give rise to abnormal gross and fine motor skills that could affect a child's ability to speak, sign, or fingerspell. They may also accompany or give rise to other psychological deficits that affect learning. It is important therefore, that professional educators, audiologists, and speech pathologists become able to recognize, evaluate, and provide appropriate remediation for the range of additional problems that are to be found among children who are hearing-impaired, whether these problems are psychoneurological disabilities or whether they reflect sensory impairment or deprivation (Fig 8-5).

However, when psychoneurological or behavioral problems are manifested, they hinder the educational process of the child who is hearing-impaired regardless of the mode of education employed. As the child is monitored in an auditory-verbal communication program, there may be indications of inadequate progress in learning speech (despite aided hearing over the speech frequency range), an inability to learn the meaning of sound, poor memory and recall, failure to develop symbolic rela-

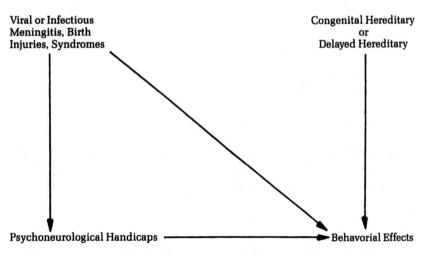

Fig 8-5.—Interrelationships of causative hearing loss with psychoneurological and behavioral effects occurring in some SNHL patients.

tionships, or inconsistent responses to sounds that should be audible. Visual problems may also hinder the learning of signs in a total communication program. Of course, if visual deficiency is corrected through refraction, it is not considered a visual disability. However, visual problems to note include poor visual recognition and memory, ocular pursuit movements, or the inability of the eyes to confluently and smoothly follow an object across the field of vision. The latter finding would indicate neurological deficit due to damage to the ocular pathways.

An extensive list of psychoneurological and psychosocial disabilities has been listed by Pollack.[26] Only a brief discussion of these will be undertaken herein in an effort to alert the educator and clinician to them.

Psychoeurological Disabilities

Psychoneurological difficulties often associated with hearing impairment include learning disabilities, apraxia or dyspraxia, dysarthria, and postural insecurity secondary to muscle tone or coordination problems. Vestibular damage must be evaluated for postural gait deficits. Poor muscular coordination in early childhood results in clumsiness, stumbling, falling, sitting difficulties, and problems with head control.[27,28] These manifestations typically indicate vestibular dysfunction. Signs of neurological deficits from brain damage include specific findings involving fine movements used in grasping, generalized muscular dysfunction, such as spasticity or flaccidity, as well as muscle contractions or chorealike contractions and tremors that may involve the "speech" muscles.

Behavioral Effects

Hyperactivity, short attention span, stress, anxiety, and inappropriate emotional responses are symptoms of the possible behavioral effects of SNHL. These symptoms probably represent a complex known as the "hyperactivity syndrome," or "attention deficit disorder."[29] Although most children with SNHL and hyperactivity show no evidence of neuropathology, some children with the behavioral dysfunction also have equivocal signs involving minor abnormalities of reflexes and tone but, above all, disorders of sensorimotor coordination.[30] In addition to the symptoms mentioned, there appears to be a high incidence of clumsiness, difficulty in left-right discrimination, dysgraphia, and generalized coordination difficulties.

Numerous attempts have been made to define the causes of hyperactivity in children with normal hearing. Some of the causes that have been suggested are genetic contribution, alcoholism in one or both parents, psychosocial disorders in parents,[31] drug use in pregnancy,[28] neonatal birth injuries,[32,33] and food additives. However, the specific nature of the problem in children with normal hearing and in those who are hearing impaired is usually unknown. A contributing factor for the child who is hearing-impaired may be the fact that auditory deprivation increases visual motivation. That is, the child who is hearing-deprived may learn to explore his or her environment visually more effectively than would otherwise have been the case.

Care must be taken in making the diagnosis of hyperactivity in a child with hearing impairment, as there is lack of specificity of the symptoms and varying degrees of overactivity. Some children just tend to be "too active."

Psychological Testing

Many nonverbal testing techniques have been designed for use with children who are hearing-impaired. Psychologists are now, therefore, generally able to assess such children's intellectual functioning and cognitive development, as well as the psychoneurological and behavioral difficulties associated with SNHL. A complete psychological evaluation of a child who is hearing-impaired should, typically, include a measurement of intelligence, an evaluation of personality structure, appraisal for brain damage, a measure of educational achievement, and an assessment of communication skills.[34]

Vernon[34] has described the tests employed by psychologists in evaluating children who are hearing-impaired. He has also reported on evaluations of each of them. The reasons for discrepancies in test results vary from one test to another and also from child to child because those with limited verbal skills may be unable to follow directions with ease. High levels of testing skill are therefore required in order to determine a child's true abilities. Some psychologists find it necessary to use two or more test batteries for each evaluation in order to obtain valid results. Psychological testing can provide not only data on intellectual performance, but also measure academic functioning and identify specific problem areas. The results of psychological testing can provide information that is of vital importance in the task of mainstreaming a child effectively.[35]

Intelligence

In the absence of concomitant neurological disorders, children who are hearing-impaired vary in intelligence from slow to gifted just as do normally hearing children. It is important that the intelligence of a child who is hearing-impaired, and his or her potential for developing communicative skills, be evaluated competently and educational goals be set realistically.

The psycholinguistic abilities of children who are normally hearing and mentally retarded are adversely affected. Rohr and Burr[36] compared the psycholinguistic abilities of 131 children who were mentally retarded (IQs of 30 to 60) in different etiological classifications that included Down's syndrome, biologically brain damaged (LBW and congenital conditions, such as microcephaly), environmentally caused retardation (birth injury, postnatal head injury), and those of unknown causes. The Down's syndrome children had significantly lower verbal-auditory abilities than did the children in other mental retardation etiological groups. Although children in all etiological classifications had a deficit in auditory sequential memory, the specific psycholinguistic processes studied by the authors included auditory reception, auditory association, verbal expression, auditory memory, and grammatical closure.

Treatment

The many problems and needs of children with SNHL who have psychoneurological disabilities and behavioral deficits often require a management program that includes antihyperactivity medication, individual educational instruction, and occupational and psychological therapy. In the case of hyperactivity, the use of stimulants alone has not been considered a successful therapeutic regimen[4] and is only of symptomatic value. The treatment of hyperactivity with various diets has become popular with some professionals, school personnel, and parents in recent years. The dietary considerations most often given attention with this treatment include food additives, food allergies, sugar intolerance, megavitamins, and trace mineral excesses or deficiencies. Although such dietary restrictions are thought not to be harmful to children, examination of this therapeutic approach has revealed improvement in 10% or fewer of the patients.[37] The creative educator can institute therapy by persistently increasing the child's attention span through the use of varied and interesting methods.

Explicitly, certain muscle incoordination problems resulting from vestibular dysfunction or brain damage will impede progress in learning activities in any program. The role of the physical and occupational therapists is to evaluate and treat such disabilities by altering neural dysfunction through enhancement of the central activity of the motor and sensory systems,[1] and the functional development of the tactile, perceptive, vestibular, and visual systems.

Counseling or psychological habilitation should be provided for the child and the family. Preferably, psychological monitoring should be a routine matter. Unfortunately, it often takes a bit of adversity, such as the suspicion of mental retardation or lack of expected progress in the program, to pull these professionals together as an educational team.

Scope of Treatment

The advantage to the educator, audiologist, and speech pathologist of knowing the diagnosis, or the cause of the hearing loss, should be reemphasized, for it enables them to better evaluate and anticipate associated psychological problems.

Viral causes of SNHL (rubella and CMV infection) have been known in some cases to result in mental retardation.[38,39] The virus may affect the CNS in addition to the labyrinth. Birth injuries and manifestations of LBW (asphyxia and hyperbilirubinemia) are known pathologically to cause damage to brain nuclei,[40] and meningitis has been shown to cause CNS damage at the cellular level.[41,42] It must be stressed that children in this group who are slow learners should not be labeled as being mentally deficient. However, these children will have a higher incidence of psychoneurological disabilities (ECHO Foundation statistics) and resultant behavioral effects. Psychological testing is usually indicated in these cases, especially if mental retardation or brain injury is suspected. Specialized programs should be provided when indicated for some of the children in this group. The educational modality may need to be changed from auditory to visual-auditory to total communication. If the child has been mainstreamed, the most effective training may require specialized programs.

Vestibular damage frequently occurs in children affected by meningitis, CMV infection, and some hereditary syndromes; obvious developmental lags are common. It is not unusual for such children to have both SNHL and gross developmental disorders. In many instances, however, the incoordination will resolve in time; if not, remediation using occupational therapy is advised.

Children with SNHL from congenital hereditary or delayed hereditary causes and without signs of an associated syndrome tend not to have psychoneurological disabilities. Behavioral defects are more common in this group. However, learning disabilities may be manifested, just as they are in children with typical hearing.

Although this "classification" of CNS and peripheral nervous system deficits may seem to be a categorization, it is merely a logical ordering (Fig 8–5). Each infant or child with an SNHL, regardless of the diagnosis, is unique. Even when different children with SNHL due to meningitis are compared, findings differ and each child has an individual manifestation of his or her condition. Such is the mechanism of damage that occurs with CNS or peripheral nervous system disorders. Yet, when the diagnosis of SNHL is known, these affective disorders can be predicted and even anticipated.

The acquisition of language skills is not a specific neurological entity. Rather, it is a psychological manifestation of an exclusive sensory processing skill. Although the psychologist is capable of identifying and treating abnormal psychoneurological and psychosocial deficits, there is no method available to determine which child with SNHL has the capability of learning speech and language or the extent to which children without oral skills will approach cognitive development (Fig 8–6).

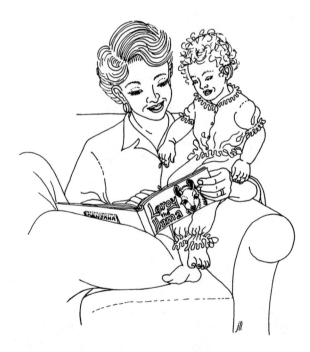

Fig 8-6.—Most children who are hearing-impaired have the potential to learn to talk, and most mothers, like this one who is reading to her child, can provide optimal opportunities for them to do so.

REFERENCES

1. Ling D. *Early Intervention for Hearing-impaired Children: Total Communication.* San Diego, Ca: College-Hill Press; 1984:5.
2. Duchan JF. Language assessment: the pragmatics revolution. In: Naremore RC, ed. *Language Science: Recent Advances.* San Diego, Ca: College-Hill Press; 1984.
3. Fischer RM. Habilitation of the hearing-impaired child. In: Jerger J, ed. *Pediatric Audiology: Current Trends.* San Diego, Ca: College-Hill Press; 1984: 177-202.
4. Deno EL. Special education as developmental capital. *Exceptional Children* 1970;37:229-240.
5. Ling D, Milne M. The development of speech in hearing-impaired children. In: *Amplification in Education.* Washington, DC: Alexander Graham Bell Association for the Deaf; 1981:98-108.
6. Ling D. The integration of speech and language training. Unpublished paper presented at the International Congress in Education of the Deaf, Hamburg, Germany, August 1980.
7. Ling D. The education of hearing-impaired children. *Public Health Rev.* 1975;4:135.
8. Ling D. *The Foundations of Spoken Language for Hearing-Impaired Children.* Washington, DC: Alexander Graham Bell Association for the Deaf; 1989.
9. Griffey MN. A survey of present methods of developing language in deaf children. In: Mulholland AM, ed. *Oral Education Today and Tomorrow.* Washington, DC, Alexander Graham Bell Association for the Deaf; 1981:119-131.
10. Bell AG. *The Mechanism of Speech.* New York, NY: Funk and Wagnells, 1916.
11. Perigoe CB, Ling D. Generalization of speech skills in hearing-impaired children. *Volta Review.* 1986;88:351-366.
12. Ling D, Ling AH. *Aural Habilitation: The Foundations of Verbal Learning.* Washington, DC: Alexander Graham Bell Association for the Deaf; 1978:144-146.
13. Sherrick, CE. Basic and applied research on tactile aids for deaf people: progress and prospects. *Acoustical Society of America.* 1984;78:78-83.
14. Weisenberger J. Tactile aids for speech perception and production by hearing-impaired people. *Volta Review.* 1989;91(5):79-100.
15. Cornett RO. Cued Speech. *American Annals of the Deaf.* 1967;112:3-13.
16. Cornett RO, Daisey ME. *The Cued Speech Resource Book.* Raleigh, Nc: The National Cued Speech Association; 1992:17-27.
17. Bonet JP. *The limitations of writing and pictures for teaching the deaf to speak* (in Spanish). Madrid: Par Francisco Arbaco de Angelo; 1620.
18. Bender R. *The Conquest of Deafness.* Cleveland; Oh: Case Western Reserve University; 1970.
19. Lynas W. *Communication Options in the Education of Deaf Children.* London: Whurr Publishers, Ltd; 1994.
20. Bornstein HA. A description of some current sign systems designed to represent English. *Am Ann Deaf.* 1973;118:454-463.

21. Wolk S, Schildroth AN. Deaf children and speech intelligibility. In: Schildroth AN, Karchmer MA, eds. *Deaf Children in America.* San Diego, Ca: College-Hill Press; 1986;139-156.

22. Anthony DA associates, eds. *Seeing Essential English.* Anaheim, Ca; Educational Services Division, Anaheim Union High School District; 1971:1,2.

23. Gustason G, Pfetzing D, Zaqolkow E. *Signing Exact English.* Rossmoor, Ca: Modern Signs Press; 1972.

24. Johnson RE, Liddell SK, Erting CJ. Unlocking the curriculum: principles for achieving access in deaf education. *Gallaudet Research Institute Working Paper.* Washington,DC: Gallaudet University; 1989;89:3.

25. Karchmer MA, Kirwin LA. *The Use of Hearing Aids by Hearing Impaired Students in the United States.* Washington, DC: office of Demographic Studies, Gallaudet College; 1977.

26. Pollack D. *Educational Audiology for the Limited Hearing Infant and Preschooler.* Springfield, Il: Charles C. Thomas; 1985.

27. Rapin I. Hypoactive labyrinths and motor development. *Clin Pediatr.* 1974;13:922-937.

28. Eviatar L, Eviatar A. Development of head control and vestibular responses in infants treated with aminoglycoside. *Dev Med Child Neurol.* 1982;24: 372-379.

29. Varley CK. Attention deficit disorder (the hyperactivity syndrome): a review of selected issues. *Dev Behav Pediatr.* 1984;5:254-258.

30. Werry JS, Aman MG. The reliability and diagnostic validity of the physical and neurological examination for soft signs (PANESS). *J Autism Child Schizo.*1976;6:253-262.

31. Cantwell DP. Psychiatric illness in the families of hyperactive children. *Arch Gen Psychiatry.* 1972;27:414-417.

32. Werner EE, Smith RS. *Kauai's Children Come of Age.* Honolulu, Hi: University Press of Hawaii; 1977.

33. Sammeroff A, Chandler M. Reproductive risk in the continuum of caretaking casualties. In: Horowitz F, ed. *Review of Child Development Research.* Chicago, Il: University of Chicago Press; 1975.

34. Vernon M. The psychological examination. In: Berg FS, Fletcher SG, eds. *The Hard of Hearing Child.* New York: Grune & Stratton; 1970:217-231.

35. Fischer RM. Habilitation of the hearing-impaired child. In: Jerger J, ed. *Pediatric Audiology: Current Trends.* San Diego, Ca: College-Hill Press, 1984: 177-202.

36. Rohr A, Burr DB. Etiological differences in patterns of psycholinguistic development of children of IQ 30 to 60. *Am J Ment Defic.* 1978;82:549-553.

37. Varley CK. Diet and the behavior of children with attention deficit disorders. *J Am Acad Child Psychiatry.* 1984;23:182-185.

38. Pass RF, Stagno S, Myers GJ, Alford CA. Outcome of symptomatic congenital CMV infection: results of long-term longitudinal follow-up. *Pediatrics.* 1980; 66:758-762.

39. Barr B, Lundstrom R. Deafness following maternal rubella. *Acta Otolaryngol.* 1961;53:413-423.

40. Ahdab-Barmada M. Neonatal kernicterus: neuropathologic diagnosis. In: Levine RL, Maisels MJ, eds. *Hyperbilirubinemia in the Newborn*. Report of the 85th Ross Conference on Pediatric Research. Columbus, Oh: Ross Laboratories; 1983:2-10.
41. Fishman RA, Sligar K, Hake RB. Effects of leukocytes on brain meatabolism in granulocytic brain edema. *Ann Neurol*. 1977;2:89-94.
42. Fishman RA. Brain edema. *N Engl J Med*. 1975;193:706-711.

CHAPTER

Cochlear Implants

Dennis G. Pappas Jr, MD

Education never ends, Watson. It is a series of lessons.
The Adventure of The Red Circle
Sherlock Holmes

To understand the function of a cochlear implant, one must first understand the function of the cochlea. As described in Chapter 1, the cochlea's function is to convert sound energy into electrochemical signals that are meaningful to the auditory cortex of the brain. Sensorineural deafness typically involves the loss of hair cells of the organ of Corti within the cochlea. Proximal neural elements (auditory nerve and central auditory pathways) to some extent or number, typically survive and can therefore be stimulated. The cochlear implant serves to bypass the damaged or absent hair cells, taking advantage of the surviving auditory elements.

Should there be a totally nonfunctioning acoustic nerve or retrocochlear pathology (brainstem or cortical), a cochlear implant will not be of assistance in improving the hearing signals of the deaf person. If the cochlear nerve is nonfunctional, newer implants called "brainstem implants" offer hope of improving hearing thresholds. No technology today can improve hearing if the source of deafness lies at the level of the cerebral cortex.

In essence, hearing aids amplify sound to the cochlea. Cochlear implants replace the cochlea. Hearing aids rely on existing hair cells. Implants replace hair cells. Implants restore the sensation of hearing, whereas hearing aids exploit existing hearing.

In adults, acquired causes of profound and total hearing loss include bilateral Ménière's disease, use of ototoxic drugs, syphilis, cochlear otosclerosis, head injury, and a group of cases in which the etiology is unknown, including those with viral causes. The cause can be determined in approximately 70% of children with hearing loss.[1] Congenital causes include those that are hereditary (recessively and dominantly inherited syndromes) and congenitally acquired (birth injuries, viral, meningitis). Acquired hearing loss in children is most commonly due to meningitis. Other causes may include those mentioned previously for adults.

Although it has not been proved, the most receptive cochlear implant patient will probably be the one with the largest number and greatest distribution of surviving eighth nerve fibers. Reports from several studies of the temporal bone from SNHL patients are available in most of the mentioned etiological categories and give information regarding the distribution of nerve fibers. Spiral ganglion populations have been reported as good in some cases of genetically based types of congenital SNHL, temporal bone fractures, Ménière's disease, and ototoxicity.[2-4] Populations of nerve fibers were found to be diminished in cases of bacterial labyrinthitis, meningitis, and congenital syphilis; somewhat intermediate numbers were found in otosclerosis and dysplasia of the cochlea.[4]

The type of hearing impairment resulting from complications of birth injuries or viral infections may involve sensory and neural components of the auditory system or central nuclei. With hearing loss due to hyperbilirubinemia or anoxia, neuropathological studies have disclosed lesions in the cochlear nuclei.[5-7] On the other hand, neurophysiological tests have supported the auditory nerve as the site-of-lesion for hearing impairment due to birth injury.[8]

Regardless of the lesion causing hearing loss, there is strong evidence of the high prevalence of brain damage among patients who had suffered birth injury.[9,10] Neuropathological studies have demonstrated brain damage in various locations as a basis for neurological manifestations other than hearing loss.[11] Furthermore, psychodiagnostic evidence of CNS dysfunction tends to emerge to explain why educational achievement is hindered. These psychoneurological and psychosocial disabilities have already been discussed.

Psychological disabilities that impede learning are often related to etiological factors. From the interrelationship of these two, it is clear that understanding the problems of the individual with hearing loss requires a fundamental knowledge of the process of hearing and the nature of the deprivation. When cochlear implants are used, awareness of the distinct patterns in language deficiency manifested in different etiological categories could be beneficial in planning language training programs to meet the specific needs of individual.

HISTORICAL OVERVIEW OF COCHLEAR IMPLANTS

Habilitation and rehabilitation of a large portion of individuals who are hearing-impaired was greatly enhanced by providing increased power and miniaturization in hearing aids. For those with a hearing loss so profound that hearing aids offer little or no benefit, the cochlear implant holds promise. The theorem of that device dates back several centuries to the noninvasive experiments of Count Alexandro Volta and others.

Beginning the modern era of cochlear implantation, the French scientists André Djourno, Charles Eyriès, and Bernard Vallancien introduced the possibilities for this revolutionary device in 1957. Djourno and colleagues published results of successful stimulation of the cochlear nerve in two human subjects. However, technical difficulties discouraged this group from continuing their research.[12]

From 1964 to 1966, F. Blair Simmons and colleagues from Stanford University Medical School reported results of direct electrical stimulation of the cochlear nerve and inferior colliculus in a patient undergoing a craniectomy for a cerebellar ependymoma. This stimulation of the brain (inferior colliculus) produced no hearing acuity. More extensive studies were reported by Simmons et al.[13] Six electrodes were implanted into the modiolus of the cochlea in a patient with total SNHL. With these electrodes, nerve fibers of different frequencies could be stimulated. Their work showed that a few microamperes of current stimulated the eighth cranial nerve sufficiently to produce an auditory sensation that increased in loudness with increased current amplitude. Since both electrode selection and the repetition rate of the stimulus both affected the tone, it was reasonable to conclude that two methods of encoding tones were operating within one group of auditory fibers.

Skepticism of the medical community, and especially peers in California, about the benefits of an implant to electrically stimulate the cochlea was prevalent and persistent during this time. Indeed, some of the basic scientists expressed open hostility. The failure of this procedure to gain credibility was due primarily to ill-advised and poorly controlled publicity in which the device was reported to provide understanding of speech, ability to converse over the telephone, hear birds singing, and enjoy music, among other extravagant claims.

Simmons and his colleagues discontinued this project because of associated complications, such as CSF leakage, and because the anticipated benefit was not promising over time. Prior to Simmon's work, House, Doyle, and Doyle experienced similar discouraging results with an implanted electrode system.[14]

The 1968 work of Michelson was pivotal in the development of the cochlear implant, for it produced the first favorable results from this procedure.[15] His animal studies, which demonstrated that intracochlear electrodes were functional over long periods of time, were followed by his report of electrically stimulating the cochlea in four human patients.

In May 1971, Michelson reported his experience using the single channel implant in humans at the American Otologic Society meeting in San Francisco. He further documented his historic achievement, the first successful series of single channel cochlear implants in humans, in the *Annals of Otology, Rhinology, and Laryngology*.[16]

Michelson's presentation before the American Otological Society generated lively dialogue among the four discussants during which Lurie's rebuttal included the observation that if it was true, it would be the first time in history anyone has heard without a cochlea! His skepticism was shared by two of the other discussants. House, who had implanted three patients (unreported) at the time, was the fourth member of the group, and the sole believer in Michelson's premise and results. By that time, House had already promoted a surgical procedure (through the mastoid to the round window via the facial recess) that prevented the complications that accompanied transcanal electrode placement.

House had also begun compiling a list of potential implant candidates in 1962. One of his first volunteers was a young man who had suffered a complete hearing loss following lifesaving antibiotic therapy several years previously. Six years later, at the age of 39, he underwent the first stimulation tests, and on June 18, 1970, an implant was placed in his right ear. Extensive postimplant studies of this patient over a 2-year period guided the engineering development of the first "take-home" stimulator package.

From 1973 through 1979, important events occurred in the area of cochlear implantation; the device was implanted in a large number of patients, animal research projects grew in number and scope, and postimplant evaluation was undertaken ("the Pittsburgh study"). In 1979, House held a training course for the use of the single channel implant in Los Angeles. The purpose of this course was to train and organize a team of approximately 20 co-investigators throughout the United States in a multi-center study of the House cochlear implant in adults. Each otologist-participant was required to bring a complete cochlear implant team, including an audiologist and a psychologist. By assimilating the information supplied by them, House was able to construct a broad base from which to proceed. From this meeting he devised the clinical pattern for cochlear implant evaluations, including audiological and psychological assessments, that remains dominant today.

During the same period that House and his group in Los Angeles were working towards their objectives, Graeme M. Clarke and his group at the University of Melbourne, in Australia, developed a multichannel prototype receiver in 1978. The first two implantations with this device occurred in 1978 and 1979.[17] Clarke's 1981 report was the second account of a cochlear implant providing useful speech discrimination based on preliminary results with the earliest Nucleus multichannel device. The first implant approved for open market was the 3M/House single channel version in 1984.

Other implant devices have been marketed in the intervening years since Michelson's initial report, but none differed appreciably from, nor were as significant, as those mentioned. Presently, the most commonly used cochlear implants are two multichannel designs, the Nucleus 22 channel and the Clarion, introduced by the University of California in San Francisco. The Ineraid (the prototype of the Utah Groups in the mid-1970s) is no longer available. A single channel design has been reintroduced by House. Multichannel implants have demonstrated improvements in speech perception and understanding. Other implants have been introduced in Europe.

SELECTION

First, inappropriate selection, loudness levels, or defective hearing aids must be addressed. Inappropriate amplification is commonly a problem regardless of the level of hearing impairment. Modification or replacement of children's hearing aids should be the first step in the process of evaluation for the cochlear implant (CI) or for the learning program. According to Daniel Ling, to the skilled listener the child with an inappropriate hearing aid will reveal inappropriate speech patterns in many ways when their hearing aids are failing them (Washington Regional Conference for Auditory-Verbal International [AVI], 9/29/96). Ling felt that only a small proportion of children who have problems with inappropriate amplification are candidates for cochlear implants.

When appropriate hearing aids are inadequate, typically only in children with total or near total deafness for a significant range of speech sources, these children are candidates for CIs. Such a child with a profound hearing loss, successfully fitted with a CI and well-mapped, should receive speech signals for the natural acquisition of spoken language. Thus, the child with an implant should easily receive speech signals comparable to that of a moderate hearing loss child using appropriate aids.

For those who need CIs, the earlier in life they receive them, the better. Ling has observed superior speech discrimination and spoken language skills among children who received them in early infancy as compared with those who, though equally hearing-impaired from early infancy, received implants in later childhood (Washington Regional Conference for AVI, 9/29/96). This is one reason implantation should not be postponed while waiting for improved technology.

Due to temporal bone growth and development, children under age 2 have not, as yet, received implants. Age and hearing qualifications are only a small part of the implantation process. Postoperative compliance is of utmost importance in children. The family plays a huge role in success, whereas with adults this is not necessarily so.

IMPLANTS AVAILABLE

Two multichannel cochlear implant systems are commonly in use in the United States. Both the Nucleus and the Clarion implant have been approved for children. The Med-El, Laura, and MXM systems are available in Europe. There are factors that influence the effectiveness of cochlear implant systems such as the number and location of activated electrodes, the method of current transmission, the stimulation rate, and the speech coding strategy (Table 9–1). It is worthwhile to understand the

Table 9–I. Characteristics of Cochlear Implant Devices

CIS*	Med-EI	Clarion	Laura	MXM	Nucleus
Information	Full Spectrum	Full Spectrum	Full Spectrum	FFT	Maximal Peaks
RATE per ave.channel	Max 18 000 1500	Max 6667 833	Max 12 500 1500	4500 145-400, FO	Max 1500 250
Actual Channels	12	8 mono-/	8 mono-/	15 com.	3-10: ave 6
Per stimulation cycle	monopopolar	bipolar	bipolar	ground	bipolar; com.ground
Electrode	24 + ground	16 + ground	16 + ground	15 + ground	22 contacts
Electrode spacing	2.6mm	2.0mm	2.05mm	0.70mm	0.75mm
Telemetry	Yes	Yes	Yes	No	No
CIS strategy	Yes	Adapted	Adapted	No	No
Stored Programs	3	3	1	2	1

Note. Update information. It was reported that the Nucleus C124M is capable of providing a CIS strategy which is specified to stimulate at a maximum overall rate of ca. 15 000 pps on 12 channels. The implant has telemetry capability and adds a monopolar configuration. The associated speech processor has a capacity for four stored programs. Overview of the five major cochlear implant systmes.

Taken from D.J. Allum[18] with permission.

* CIS (Continuous Interlearned Sampler)

differences between implant devices, and these features have been elucidated many times in the literature, most recently by Allum.[18] There is variance in the responses of implants, though these differences are not yet available in the scientific literature.

REHABILITATION

Information and Support

It is of importance to explain the mode of operation of the implant components, the batteries and their recharging characteristics, and number of hours of recommended use.

It should also be explained to the patient that he or she has individual involvement aside from that of the clinical rehabilitation process. Patients need to alertly seek environmental sounds, such as house and street noises; they are advised to participate in conversations with family and friends; to watch television; and especially encouraged to avoid withdrawing into isolation.

PROGNOSIS

Though not scientifically documented, there are educated observations regarding various implanted groups. One observation is that older children or adults switching from hearing aids to CIs maintain habitual traits involving speech misperceptions and misproductions. A second observation is that those children that return to a predominately manual or total communication program are not focused on improvement of both listening and speech skills; therefore, the performance of these children is limited.

The NIH consensus statement on CIs in adults and children (1995) points out that there is a variance in improvement in speech perception and production in children following cochlear implantation. The variance, they stated, depends on age of onset, age of implantation, the nature and intensity of rehabilitation, and the mode of communication.[19]

Implants allow a wonderful range of sounds at all frequencies. A child with a "corner configuration" that does not elicit sound at 4k will not learn soft sibilant sounds with the most powerful amplification for hearing aids, but may hear and learn the "s" sound with a CI.

ETHICAL CONSIDERATIONS

Persons who are hearing-impaired and their advocates, like society in general, are torn by schisms and form subgroups. While no one method of teaching children who are hearing-impaired can possibly meet each individual need, each subgroup, frequently without due consideration of the individual differences that exist among those who are hearing-impaired, seeks to promote educational programs that reflect its own preferred form of communication. The concepts underlying the various views as to what is best for all children who are hearing-impaired have emerged as persons who are hearing-impaired and other minority groups have come to achieve political significance. Persons who are hearing-impaired, in much the same way as other minority groups, seek to achieve their goals through promoting public awareness of their needs and special interests. Those who advocate sign language, the *culturally Deaf*, have become a highly visible force proclaiming the pride, power, and culture of their particular group. Those who speak, like former Miss America Heather Whitestone, may have much worse hearing than many who are culturally Deaf, but they are, as a rule, a much less visible minority. This is because people do not recognize speakers who are hearing-impaired as essentially different from themselves, particularly as speakers tend to integrate effectively into the mainstream of society. Individuals who are hearing-impaired, such as Heather Whitestone, see oral communication as the main tool for integrating into the hearing world. There is, therefore, less social isolation of members of this group.

COST

Cost for a CI varies from area to area. In the United States, the Nucleus implant costs $18 000. There is also the expense of the hospital (operating room), surgeons' fees (preop evaluation and fee of surgery), and rehabilitation.

Individuals needing CIs are at a noted economic disadvantage. Studies that evaluate the benefit of implants in children in relation to cost are important in analyzing such economic disadvantages.[20]

CI cost is covered by many insurance plans in the United States. There is a tendency for some managed care plans to exclude or reimburse at a low rate, a practice that will limit the social and vocational opportunities of the individuals who are profoundly deaf.

EVALUATION FOR CANDIDACY

The preimplant evaluation involves preliminary medical and audiological evaluations which may take several months to complete. The preliminary testing will determine if the patient meets general candidacy requirements.

The appropriate candidate for cochlear implantation has a profound hearing loss and receives little or no benefit from the most powerful hearing aids. No benefit with hearing aids can be defined as the inability to identify words from a closed set of choices.

During the evaluation period, the patient will be fitted with a hearing aid if an appropriate aid is not currently being worn. After an adequate trial period of approximately 3 to 6 months, testing will be conducted to determine if the hearing aid can provide useful hearing perception.

SURGICAL PROCEDURE

Surgery is required to insert the internal coil and electrodes. The incision used is not that of a typical mastoidectomy. Instead, the incision is extended posteriorly to prevent contact between the internal coil of the implant and the skin edges of the incision. Internal coil "eyeball fittings" are made in the outer table of the skull behind the upper portion of the ear, adjacent to the helix. Special burrs are used to form a circular seat in the temporal bone for secure placement of the coil immediately into the circular seat. Tunnels are made in the temporal bone to anchor sutures that will hold the internal coil in position.

Below the internal coil, and immediately behind the ear, a simple mastoidectomy is done with exposure and identification of most of the important structures of the mastoid. The facial recess, an area between the bony external auditory canal and the bony covering of the facial nerve, is removed to expose the round window in the middle ear.[21] The bony lip of the round window is then removed, and the true membrane of the window is identified. The bony partition of the inferior portion of the round window is thinned just adjacent to the sulcus of the membrane. The active electrodes are placed approximately 6 mm into the scala tympani through an opening in the inferior portion of the round window. Temporalis fascia, taken from the superior area skin incision, is then inserted around the round window for support of the active electrode. Another piece of fascia is placed in the facial recess. The entire surgical procedure takes no longer than 1.5 hours.

RISKS OF IMPLANTS

The risks generally associated with mastoid surgery (anesthesia complications, infection, and facial nerve injury) have been minimal. There have been incidental reports of meningitis, CSF leaks, imbalance, facial nerve spasm, or facial nerve paralysis as a result of the implant procedure. In children who have received a CI, there has been no associated problem of otitis media or the spread of otitis media into the inner ear, nor have any neurological or psychological complications emerged.

Typically, the most common complication of cochlear implantation is flap breakdown with exposure or partial extrusion of the internal coil.

COCHLEAR IMPLANTATION IN CHILDREN

The effectiveness of the CI in children has been proven successful. An immediate feature demonstrated by the implanted child is that of listening followed by speech production. Typically, it takes 2 to 3 years following implantation to integrate useful information that develops as a child's spoken language acquisition.

For the patient who became deaf postlingually, rehabilitation is usually shorter. This is especially true if deafness was of a short duration, if the patient had an active sociocultural environment, and if good motivation is present.

RESULTS

Multichannel cochlear implants have proven safe and effective in the treatment of profound deafness. Although a wide range of results occur, the age of deafness onset has long been considered an important variable in achieving success. Postlingual deafened adults and children typically adapt to CIs more quickly and achieve open-set speech discrimination earlier than prelingual deafened patients. Yet, as implanted prelingual deafened children are followed over time, performance has continued to improve and approach the success obtained in postlingual cases as illustrated by the studies below.

Waltzman[22] and colleagues at New York University recently reported a study of 38 children who were congenitally deaf and were followed from 1 to 5 years after implantation with the Nucleus multichannel device. All subjects were implanted below the age of 5 years, and 29 children were either originally or ultimately using the newer SPEAK coding strategy. All patients obtained measurable and significant open-set speech recognition. Mean speech scores continued to improve annually with a mean 5-year phonetically balanced kindergarten (PBK) score of 58%. Thirty-seven of these children use oral language as their sole means of communication. One child uses total communication and attends a regular school but requires an interpreter in the classroom.

In 1994, Gantz et al[23] reported long-term multichannel implant results on 54 children with prelingual deafness and 5 children with postlingual deafness. The postlingual group demonstrated significant improvement in open-set speech understanding within 1 year of implantation. While only 13% of the prelingual group could identify more that 4% of words at 1 year, open set speech discrimination was measured in 82% of the prelingual cases 4 years after implantation. In this study, several children with congenital deafness ultimately outperformed some of the patients with postlingual hearing loss.

Miyamoto et al[24] reported similar findings in a 1996 study involving congenitally deaf children with multichannel implants over a protracted time course. The average performance of the multichannel cochlear implant users gradually increased over time and continued to improve even after 5 years of CI use. The average scores for subjects who had used their CI for 4 years or more exceeded 40%.

In a 1995 report, Miyamoto et al[25] compared results of 24 children with multichannel implants to that of age-matched children with prelingual profound hearing losses who used conventional hearing aids. The hearing aid subjects were grouped by unaided thresholds: "gold" subjects (pure tone average of 92 dB hearing level) and "silver" subjects (pure tone average of 104 dB hearing level). The CI users' perceptual abilities increased significantly with time. After 2 months of CI use, performance of the CI and silver hearing aid groups was similar on measures of phoneme, word, and sentence recognition. After 2½ years of CI use, CI subjects' performance exceeded that of the gold group on vowel recognition and auditory-plus-visual sentence recognition measures.

The impact of deafness etiology has also been carefully studied and does not necessarily affect performance. Deafness caused by meningitis may limit the benefit of implantation when cochlear ossification or CNS complications occur. Children with congenital deafness and children with prelingual meningitic deafness achieve similar implant results when implanted before the age of 6 years.[26] Cochlear drill-out techniques have been developed for ossified cases.

Children with cochlear malformations such as Mondini's dysplasia have also been implanted. In 1996, Hoffman et al[27] reviewed the literature and reported an additional three such cases. These children all derived auditory benefit with results comparable to age-matched cases with no cochlear dysplasia.

Current data and the above studies continue to support the importance of early detection of hearing loss and prompt intervention. Although a direct relationship between surviving neural elements and performance level has not been adequately illustrated, most agree that the shorter the period of auditory deprivation, the better the implant outcome. Only through comprehensive, longitudinal studies can the full impact of cochlear implantation be assessed.

Activating the Cochlear Implant

After the incision area has healed, the patient will return to the clinic for fitting the external parts of the cochlear implant. It will be approximately 4 weeks between the surgery and the initial fitting session, frequently called the initial simulation, or tune up. Before the initial stimulation session, the implant will not provide hearing because the external parts are required for hearing.

At the initial stimulation session, the headset is fitted to the patient. Then a computer and a special computer program are used to program the patient's speech processor to produce these signals. These signals are used to determine how much sound stimulation is needed for the patient to hear sound. The speech processor is programmed for the individual's hearing needs.

During the programming session, the audiologist measures the threshold level and maximum comfort level for each electrode. These measurements are called a MAP. The threshold level is the softest level of sound that the patient can hear consistently. The maximum comfort level is the amount of stimulation which allows even the loudest sound in the environment to be heard comfortably. The electrical stimulation will be heard as different pitches and loudness levels.

Several additional programming sessions will follow in the coming weeks. During these sessions, the implant will be fine-tuned to the patient's individual needs. At each session, the audiologist will adjust the programming of the speech processor so that the patient will become comfortable with louder sounds and have improved sound quality. The additional mapping sessions are necessary because it takes time for the hearing nerve to adapt to the electrical signals and for the brain to interpret the new signals as sound.

Troubleshooting

To troubleshoot the speech processor, the following steps should be conducted in order:

1. Set the function knob to the "T" position. The microphone light will illuminate constantly if the battery is properly charged. If the "M" light blinks slowly (once per second), there may be a problem with the battery. If the "M" light continues to work improperly after a new battery is inserted the speech processor needs to be taken to the implant center for repair.
2. Set the function knob to "N" and the sensitivity knob to 4 or 5. Then place the transmitting coil against the front center of the speech processor. If the complete system is working, both the "M" and "C" (coil) lights should flash when sound is present.
3. If the "M" light stays on constantly when the function knob is in the "T" position, but does not flash when in the "N" position, the long cord should be replaced. If the "M" light still does not flicker when sound is present, go to step 4.
4. Replace the short cord (coil connecting cable). If the "M" light still does not flicker with sound present, go to step 5.
5. Replace the microphone with either a spare microphone or the lapel microphone. The problem could be with the headset microphone. The speech processor could need to be evaluated at the implant center.
6. If replacing the microphone does not correct the problem, the transmitting coil should be replaced and tested against the center of the speech processor. If the problem is not corrected with the changes, the speech processor should be taken to the implant center for repair.

CONCLUSION

The CI, which was introduced for implantation in children in 1980,[28] is the most current and innovative advancement in the habilitation of children who are hearing-impaired. The possibility of at least partial restoration of auditory function by this device provides an opportunity to develop auditory-vocal linkage in speech in a new and meaningful way.

Remediation of hearing by use of a CI is not to be considered a cure for deafness. There are many variables active in the educational area of the child who is hearing-impaired that may influence educational success.

These variables include the individual's intelligence, the intelligence and participation of the parents, socioeconomic factors, environmental interactions, psychoneurological and psychosocial disabilities, and quality of the therapeutic program. It is necessary to have a thorough knowledge of deaf children and to master a deep understanding of the device that was chosen for implantation to obtain the best results with a cochlear implant.

REFERENCES

1. Pappas DG. A study of the high risk registry for sensorineural hearing impairment. *Otolaryngol Head Neck Surg.* 1983;91:41-44.
2. Bergstrom L. Some pathologies of sensory and neural hearing loss. *Can J Otolaryngol.* 1975;(suppl 2):1-28.
3. Kerr A, Schuknecht HF. The spiral ganglion in profound deafness. *Acta Oto Laryngol.* 1968;65:586-598.
4. Otte J, Schuknecht HF, Kerr AG. Ganglion cell populations in normal and pathological human cochleae. Implications for cochlear implantation. *Laryngoscope.* 1978;88:1231-1246.
5. Goodhill V. Auditory pathway lesions resulting from Rh incompatibility. In: McConnell F, Ward PH, eds. *Deafness in Childhood.* Nashville, Tn: Vanderbilt University Press; 1967.
6. Dublin WB. *Fundamentals of Sensorineural Auditory Pathology.* Springfield Ill: Charles C Thomas; 1976:173-205.
7. Lindsay JR. Inner ear pathology in congenital deafness. *Otolaryngol Clin North Am.* 1971;4:245-290.
8. Chisin R, Perlman M, Sohmer H. Cochlear and brainstem responses in hearing loss following neonatal hyperbilirubinemia. *Ann Otol Rhinol Laryngol.* 1979;88:352-357.
9. Vernon M. Prematurity and deafness: the magnitude and nature of the problem among deaf children. *Except Child.* 1967;33:289-298.
10. Myklebust HR. The deaf child with other handicaps. *Am Ann Deaf.* 1958;103:496-509.
11. Ahdab-Barmada M. Neonatal kernicterus: neuropathologic diagnosis. In: Levine RL, Maisels MJ, eds. *Hyperbilirubinemia in the Newborn.* Report of the 85th Ross Conference on Pediatric Research. Columbus, Oh: Ross Laboratories, 1983:2-10.
12. Djourno A, Eyriés C. Prosthése auditive par excitation electrique á demeure. *Presse Med.* 1957;35:14.
13. Simmons F, Mongeon C, Lewis W, Huntington D. Electrical stimulation of acoustical nerve and inferior colliculus: results in man. *Arch Otolaryngol.* 1964;80:388–391. Epley J, Lummis R, et al. Auditory nerve: electrical stimulation in man. *Science.* 1965;148:104-106.

14. Doyle J, Doyle J, Turnbull F. Electrical stimulation of the eighth cranial nerve. *Arch. Otolaryng.* 1964;80:388-391.
15. Michelson R. Electrical stimulation of the human cochlea. Preliminary report. *Arch Otolaryngol.* 1971;93(3):317-323.
16. Michelson R. The results of electrical stimulation of the cochlea in human sensory deafness. *Ann Otol Rhinol Laryngol.* December 1971;80(6):914.
17. Clark G, Tong Y, Black R, Forster I, Patrick J, Dewhurst D. Multiple electrode cochlear implant. *J Laryngol Otol.* 1983;91:41-44.
18. Allum, DJ, ed. *Cochlear Implant Rehabilation in Children and Adults.* San Diego, Ca: Singular Publishing Group, Inc.; 1996:8.
19. Cochlear Implants in Adults and Children. NIH Consensus Statement, 1995. Bethesda, Md. May 15-17,1995;13:(2):1-30.
20. Wyatt JR, Niparko, JK. Evaluation of the benefit of the multichannel cochlear implant in children in relation to its cost. In: Allum DJ, ed. *Cochlear Implant Rehabilitation in Children and Adults.* San Diego, Ca: Singular; 1996:20-30.
21. Lewis ML. A variation in technique of facial nerve decompression. *Laryngoscope.* 1956;66:1451-1463.
22. Waltzman SB, Cohen HL, Gomolin RH, et al. Open set speech perception in congenitally deaf children using cochlear implants. Am J Otol. 1997;18: 342-349.
23. Gantz FJ, Tyler RS, Woodworth GG, et al. Results of multichannel cochlear implants in congenital and acquired prelingual deafness in children: five-year follow-up. *Am J Otol.* 1994;15(suppl 2):1-7.
24. Miyamoto RT, Kirk KI, Robbins AM, et al. Speech perception and speech production skills of children with multichannel cochlear implants. *Acta Otolaryngol* (Stockh). 1996;116:240-243.
25. Miyamoto RT, Kirk KI, Todd SL, et al. Speech perception skills of children with multichannel cochlear implants or hearing aids. *Ann Otol Rhinol Laryngol.* 1995:(suppl 166):334-337.
26. Gates G, Daly K, Dichtal WJ, et al. National Institutes of Health: Consensus Development Conference Statement: Cochlear Implants in Adults and Children. Bethesda, Md, May 1995:15-17.
27. Hoffman RA, Downey LL, Waltzman SB, et al. Cochlear implantation in children with cochlear malformations. *Am J Otol.* 1997;18:184-187.
28. Eisenberg LS, Berliner KI, Thielemeir MA, et al. Cochlear implants in children. *Ear Hear.* 1983;4:41-50.

INDEX

U

Unisensory habilitation programs,
    228–231

V

Venereal Disease Research
    Laboratory (VDRL), 100
VDRL test for syphilitic infection,
    109
Ventilation tubes, benefits of, 124–125
    complications with, 128–130
    indications for placement of, 124
    protection from water, 131
    removal of, 130–131
    surgical management, 126
    type of tube employed, 126–128
Vestibular aqueduct abnormalities,
    86–87
Vestibular damage, 245
Vestibular involvement in
    meningitis, 140
Vestibular nystagmus, beats of, 51
Vestibular system, anatomy and
    physiology of, 16–21

anatomy, 16–21
vestibulo-ocular reflex, 21
Vestibular testing
    clinical testing, 48–50
    importance of for children with
        SNHL, 49–52
    caloric testing in children, 49
    computerized rotary chair
        system, 49–52
    vestibular function in children,
        46–48
Vestibule and semicircular canals, 88
Vestibulo-ocular reflex, 21
Viral causes of SNHL, 245
Virus, definition of, 97–98
Visual reinforcement audiometry, 198
Vocalization, description of, 4–5
Vowels, definition of, 5

W

Waardenburg's syndrome, 47

X

X-linked trait, 73–74